The Ultimate Anti-Inflammatory Diet Cookbook for Beginners

2000+ Days of Easy, Step-by-Step and Flavor-Packed Recipes to Boost Immunity, Reduce Pain and Simplify Life with a 28-Day Meal Plan & Shopping Guide

HELGA GRINLEY

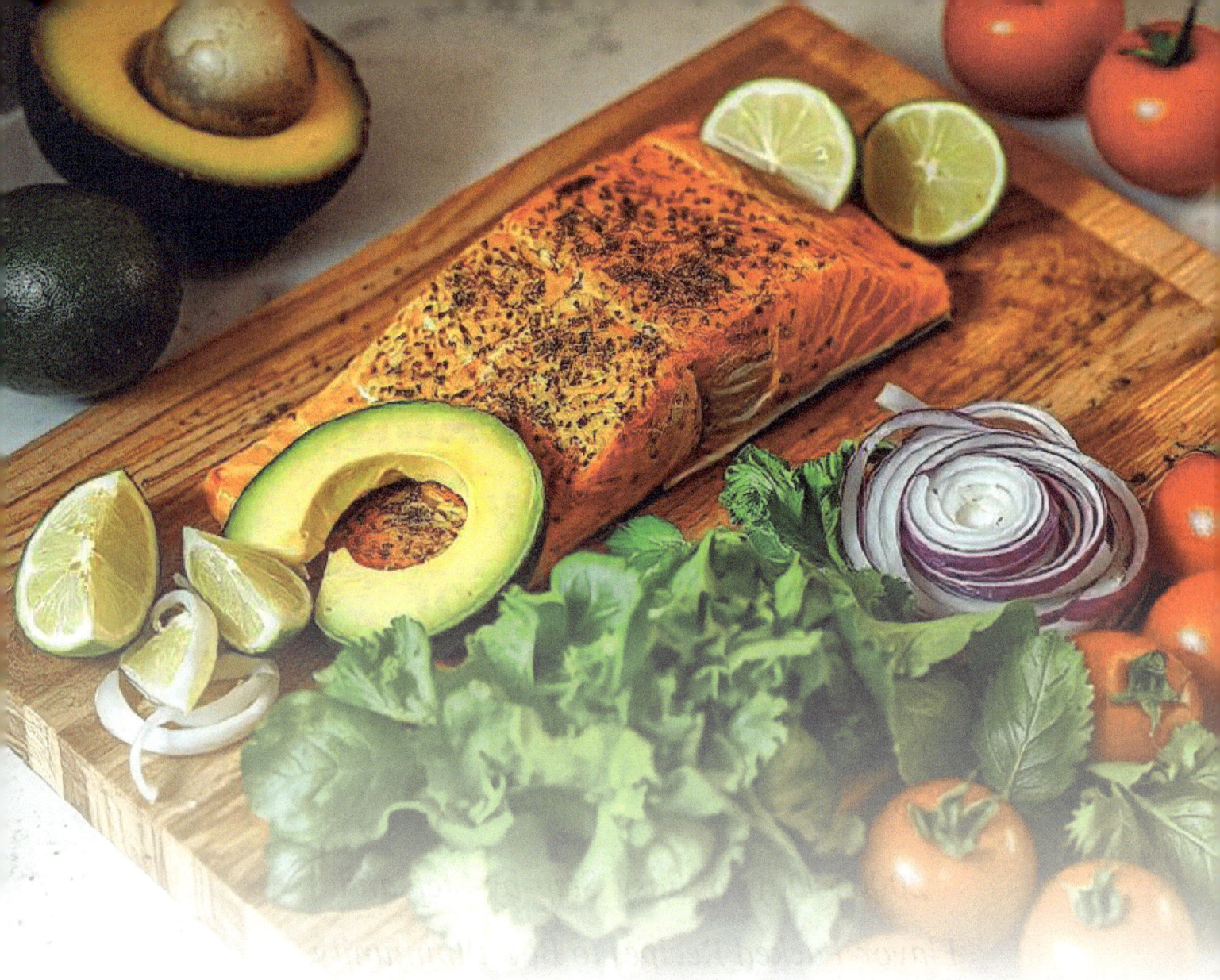

Disclaimer

The information provided in this cookbook is for general informational purposes only. It is not intended as a substitute for professional medical advice, diagnosis, or treatment. Always consult with a qualified healthcare provider before starting any diet or exercise program, particularly if you have pre-existing medical conditions or are taking medication. The author has made every effort to ensure that the information in this book is accurate and up-to-date. However, the author assumes no responsibility for errors or omissions, and no liability is assumed for damages resulting from the use of the information contained here.

CONTENTS

WELCOME TO THE ANTI-INFLAMMATORY DIET: YOUR GUIDE TO HEALTH AND WELLNESS

OVERVIEW OF INFLAMMATION AND ITS EFFECTS ON HEALTH

Inflammation is a natural response of the body to injury, infection, or harmful substances. It serves as a protective mechanism, helping to heal wounds and fight off pathogens. However, when inflammation becomes chronic, it can lead to a host of health issues. Chronic inflammation is associated with various conditions, including heart disease, diabetes, arthritis, and even certain cancers. Understanding the role of inflammation is essential for maintaining overall health.

In today's fast-paced world, many factors contribute to chronic inflammation, including poor diet, stress, lack of exercise, and exposure to environmental toxins. Recognizing the signs of inflammation, such as fatigue, joint pain, and digestive issues, is the first step toward taking control of your health.

BENEFITS OF AN ANTI-INFLAMMATORY DIET

An anti-inflammatory diet focuses on incorporating foods that help reduce inflammation in the body while eliminating those that can exacerbate it. Here are some key benefits:

• **Enhanced Immune Function**: By reducing inflammation, you can boost your immune system, helping your body fight off illnesses more effectively.

• **Reduced Pain and Discomfort**: Many people experience less joint pain and stiffness when they adopt an anti-inflammatory diet, which can improve mobility and overall quality of life.

• **Better Digestive Health**: Foods rich in fiber and probiotics can improve gut health, which is closely linked to inflammation levels in the body.

• **Improved Heart Health**: An anti-inflammatory diet often includes heart-healthy foods like fatty fish, nuts, and whole grains, which can reduce the risk of cardiovascular disease.

• **Weight Management**: This diet emphasizes whole, nutrient-dense foods that can help with weight loss and maintenance, further reducing the burden of inflammation.

• **Increased Energy Levels**: By nourishing your body with anti-inflammatory foods, you may notice an improvement in your energy levels and overall vitality.

HOW TO USE THIS COOKBOOK

Welcome to your journey toward better health with the **Anti-Inflammatory Diet for Beginners 2025**. This cookbook is designed to be your comprehensive guide to understanding and implementing an anti-inflammatory lifestyle. Here's how to make the most of it:

• **Start with the Basics**: Begin by reading through the introductory chapters that explain inflammation, its effects, and the core principles of the anti-inflammatory diet. This foundational knowledge will help you make informed choices.

• **Explore the Recipes**: Dive into the various chapters filled with easy, step-by-step recipes. Whether you're looking for breakfast ideas, hearty lunches, satisfying dinners, or healthy snacks and desserts, you'll find a wide array of options that are both delicious and nutritious.

• **Plan Your Meals**: Use the meal planning tips provided in the cookbook to create a balanced weekly menu. Planning ahead can make it easier to stick to the diet and avoid the temptation of inflammatory foods.

• **Stay Motivated**: Refer to the tips and strategies for staying motivated throughout your journey. Tracking your progress and celebrating small victories can keep you engaged and inspired.

UNDERSTANDING INFLAMMATION

WHAT IS INFLAMMATION?

Inflammation is a complex biological response that occurs when the body detects harmful stimuli, such as pathogens, damaged cells, or irritants. It is an essential part of the immune system's defense mechanism, helping to heal injuries and fight infections. It's crucial to understand the differences between acute and chronic inflammation to manage your health effectively.

ACUTE VS. CHRONIC INFLAMMATION

• **Acute Inflammation**: This type of inflammation is short-term and often arises after an injury, infection, or irritant. For instance, if you sprain your ankle, the area may become red, swollen, and painful as your body works to heal the injury. Acute inflammation typically resolves on its own once the underlying issue is addressed.

• **Chronic Inflammation**: Unlike acute inflammation, chronic inflammation persists over a longer period, sometimes for months or even years. It can result from unresolved acute inflammation or from ongoing health issues, such as autoimmune diseases, obesity, and prolonged exposure to stress. Chronic inflammation is linked to serious health conditions, including heart disease, diabetes, and certain cancers. Recognizing the signs of chronic inflammation—like fatigue, joint pain, and digestive issues—is vital for early intervention.

COMMON CAUSES AND TRIGGERS

Several factors can contribute to the development of chronic inflammation:

• **Diet**: A diet high in processed foods, refined sugars, and unhealthy fats can promote inflammation.
• **Physical Inactivity**: Lack of regular exercise can lead to weight gain and increased inflammation.
• **Stress**: Chronic stress triggers the release of inflammatory chemicals in the body.

• **Environmental Factors**: Exposure to pollutants, chemicals, and allergens can initiate inflammatory responses.
• **Infections**: Persistent infections can lead to chronic inflammation if the immune system remains activated for too long.

Understanding these triggers can help you make lifestyle changes that reduce inflammation and improve your overall health.

THE ROLE OF DIET IN INFLAMMATION

Your diet plays a critical role in managing inflammation. The foods you choose can either promote or combat inflammation in your body.

FOODS THAT PROMOTE INFLAMMATION

Certain foods are known to increase inflammation levels. Avoiding or limiting these items can be beneficial:

• **Processed Foods**: Foods high in added sugars, unhealthy fats, and preservatives can trigger inflammatory responses. Examples include sugary snacks, fast food, and processed meats.
• **Refined Carbohydrates**: White bread, pastries, and other refined grain products can lead to spikes in blood sugar and increased inflammation.

• **Fried Foods**: Cooking foods at high temperatures in unhealthy oils can create compounds that promote inflammation.
• **Excessive Alcohol**: While moderate alcohol consumption can have some health benefits, excessive intake can lead to inflammation and other health issues.

FOODS THAT FIGHT INFLAMMATION

On the other hand, incorporating anti-inflammatory foods into your diet can help reduce inflammation and promote overall wellness:

• **Fruits and Vegetables**: Berries, cherries, leafy greens, and cruciferous vegetables (like broccoli and cauliflower) are packed with antioxidants and nutrients that combat inflammation.

• **Healthy Fats**: Foods rich in omega-3 fatty acids, such as fatty fish (salmon, mackerel), nuts (walnuts, almonds), and seeds (chia seeds, flaxseeds), help reduce inflammation.

• **Whole Grains**: Brown rice, quinoa, and whole grain bread provide fiber and nutrients that support gut health and decrease inflammation.

• **Spices and Herbs**: Turmeric and ginger are powerful anti-inflammatory agents. Incorporating these into your meals can enhance flavor while benefiting your health.

• **Legumes**: Beans and lentils are high in fiber and nutrients, making them excellent choices for reducing inflammation.

GETTING STARTED

SETTING YOURSELF UP FOR SUCCESS

Embarking on an anti-inflammatory diet is a rewarding journey toward better health, but success often starts with a well-prepared kitchen. Creating an environment conducive to healthy cooking can make all the difference in your ability to stick to your new lifestyle. Here's how to set yourself up for success.

KITCHEN ESSENTIALS FOR ANTI-INFLAMMATORY COOKING

• **Quality Cookware**: Invest in good-quality pots, pans, and baking dishes. Non-toxic cookware, such as stainless steel or cast iron, can help you avoid harmful chemicals that may leach into your food.

• **Sharp Knives**: A good set of sharp knives will make meal preparation easier and more enjoyable.

• **Cutting Boards**: Have separate cutting boards for fruits, vegetables, and proteins to avoid cross-contamination. Choose boards made from wood or bamboo, as they are less likely to harbor bacteria than plastic.

• **Measuring Tools**: Accurate measuring cups and spoons will help you follow recipes more effectively, ensuring you get the right proportions of anti-inflammatory ingredients.

• **Food Processor or Blender**: A good quality blender or food processor can make preparing smoothies, sauces, and soups a breeze, allowing you to enjoy more nutritious meals with minimal effort.

• **Storage Containers**: Invest in a set of glass or BPA-free plastic storage containers for leftovers and meal prepping. This will help you stay organized and reduce food waste.

PANTRY STAPLES: ANTI-INFLAMMATORY INGREDIENTS TO STOCK

Stocking your pantry with anti-inflammatory staples will make it easier to whip up healthy meals on busy days. Here's a list of essential ingredients:

• **Whole Grains**: Brown rice, quinoa, barley, and farro are excellent sources of fiber and nutrients that can help reduce inflammation.

• **Healthy Fats**: Extra virgin olive oil, avocado oil, and coconut oil are great for cooking and drizzling over dishes. Include nuts (almonds, walnuts) and seeds (chia seeds, flaxseeds) for snacking and adding to recipes.

• **Spices and Herbs**: Turmeric, ginger, garlic, cinnamon, and cayenne pepper are powerful anti-inflammatory spices that can elevate the flavor of your meals while providing health benefits.

• **Legumes**: Stock up on lentils, chickpeas, and black beans, which are high in protein and fiber, making them perfect for salads, soups, and stews.

• **Canned and Frozen Fruits and Vegetables**: Fresh produce is ideal, but canned (look for low-sodium) and frozen options are convenient and just as nutritious. Berries, leafy greens, and cruciferous vegetables should be staples.

• **Fermented Foods**: Consider stocking fermented items like sauerkraut, kimchi, and yogurt, which contain probiotics that support gut health.

HOW TO PLAN YOUR MEALS

Planning your meals can significantly enhance your success on the anti-inflammatory diet. Here are some effective strategies to get started:

Meal Prepping Tips

• **Choose a Day for Prep**: Set aside a specific day each week for meal prepping. This could be Sunday, for example, when you can prepare several meals for the week ahead.

• **Batch Cooking**: Cook large quantities of grains, beans, and proteins. Portion them out into containers for easy access during the week.

• **Chop and Store**: Prepare vegetables by washing, peeling, and chopping them ahead of time. Store them in clear containers in the fridge to encourage healthy snacking and quick meal assembly.

• **Cook Once, Eat Twice**: Make extra portions of dinner so you can have leftovers for lunch the next day. This saves time and ensures you have nutritious options readily available.

• **Incorporate Variety**: Prepare a variety of proteins, grains, and vegetables to keep your meals interesting and balanced throughout the week.

CREATING A BALANCED ANTI-INFLAMMATORY MEAL PLAN

A well-rounded meal plan includes a mix of macronutrients and is rich in vitamins and minerals. Here's how to create one:

• **Include Plenty of Color**: Aim for a variety of colorful fruits and vegetables at each meal. The different colors typically indicate diverse nutrients and antioxidants.

• **Balance Your Plate**: Each meal should include a source of lean protein (chicken, fish, legumes), healthy fats (avocado, nuts, olive oil), and complex carbohydrates (whole grains, starchy vegetables).

• **Plan for Snacks**: Incorporate healthy snacks, such as cut-up veggies with hummus or a handful of nuts, to keep you satisfied between meals.

• **Be Flexible**: Life can be unpredictable, so allow for flexibility in your meal plan. It's okay to swap meals or adjust portions based on your hunger levels and schedule.

• **Listen to Your Body**: Pay attention to how different foods make you feel. Adjust your meal plan according to your energy levels, mood, and hunger cues.

By setting up your kitchen with the right tools and ingredients, and by planning your meals effectively, you'll create a solid foundation for success on your anti-inflammatory diet. In the upcoming chapters, we'll explore delicious recipes that embody these principles, making your journey enjoyable and fulfilling. Let's get cooking!

TABLES OF UNITS OF MEASUREMENT

Measurement	Milliliters (ml)	Fluid Ounces (fl oz)
1/8 tsp	0.6 ml	0.02 fl oz
1/4 tsp	1.25 ml	0.04 fl oz
1/2 tsp	2.5 ml	0.08 fl oz
3/4 tsp	3.75 ml	0.13 fl oz
1 tsp	5 ml	0.17 fl oz
1 1/2 tsp	7.5 ml	0.25 fl oz
2 tsp	10 ml	0.34 fl oz
2 1/2 tsp	12.5 ml	0.42 fl oz
1 tbsp	15 ml	0.5 fl oz
2 tbsp	30 ml	1 fl oz
1/4 cup	60 ml	2 fl oz
1/3 cup	80 ml	2.7 fl oz
1/2 cup	120 ml	4 fl oz
2/3 cup	160 ml	5.4 fl oz
3/4 cup	180 ml	6 fl oz
1 cup	240 ml	8 fl oz
1 1/2 cups	360 ml	12 fl oz
2 cups	480 ml	16 fl oz
3 cups	720 ml	24 fl oz
4 cups	960 ml	32 fl oz

Ounces (oz) Pounds (lb)	Grams (g)
1 oz	28 g
2 oz	57 g
3 oz	85 g
4 oz	113 g
5 oz	142 g
10 oz	283 g
14 oz	397 g
16 oz =1 lb	454 g
2 lb	907 g
3 lb	1,361 g
4 lb	1,814 g
5 lb	2,268 g

Fahrenheit (^{o}F)	Celsius (^{o}C)
225 ^{o}F	107 ^{o}C
250 ^{o}F	121 ^{o}C
275 ^{o}F	135 ^{o}C
300 ^{o}F	149 ^{o}C
325 ^{o}F	163 ^{o}C
350 ^{o}F	177 ^{o}C
375 ^{o}F	190 ^{o}C
400 ^{o}F	204 ^{o}C
425 ^{o}F	218 ^{o}C
450 ^{o}F	232 ^{o}C
475 ^{o}F	246 ^{o}C
500 ^{o}F	260 ^{o}C

1. SMOOTHIES & JUICES

MATCHA GREEN SMOOTHIE WITH SPINACH AND MANGO

Yield: 2 servings Preparation Time: 5 minutes Passive Time: None

Ingredients

> **1 cup** unsweetened almond milk (or coconut water for a lighter option)
> **1 cup** frozen mango chunks (rich in vitamin C and antioxidants)
> **1 cup** fresh spinach (anti-inflammatory and rich in iron and fiber)
> **1/2** banana (for natural sweetness and potassium)
> **1 tsp** matcha powder (antioxidant-rich green tea powder)
> **1 Tbsp** chia seeds (high in omega-3s and fiber)
> **1/4 tsp** ground ginger (optional, for additional anti-inflammatory benefits)
> **1 tsp** raw honey or maple syrup (optional, for sweetness)

Optional Add-ins:

> **1/4 cup** Greek yogurt or plant-based yogurt (for added creaminess and protein)
> **1 Tbsp** hemp seeds (for extra omega-3s and protein)

Instructions

1. **Prepare Ingredients**: Make sure the spinach is rinsed and the banana is peeled and broken into chunks for easy blending.
2. **Combine in Blender**: Add the almond milk, mango, spinach, banana, matcha powder, chia seeds, and ginger (if using) to the blender. If desired, add the yogurt or a plant-based alternative for a creamier texture.
3. **Blend Until Smooth**: Blend on high until smooth and creamy. If the smoothie is too thick, add a bit more almond milk until you reach your preferred consistency.
4. **Taste and Adjust**: Taste the smoothie and add honey or maple syrup if you prefer extra sweetness.
5. **Serve Immediately**: Pour the smoothie into two glasses and enjoy! Add toppings if desired.

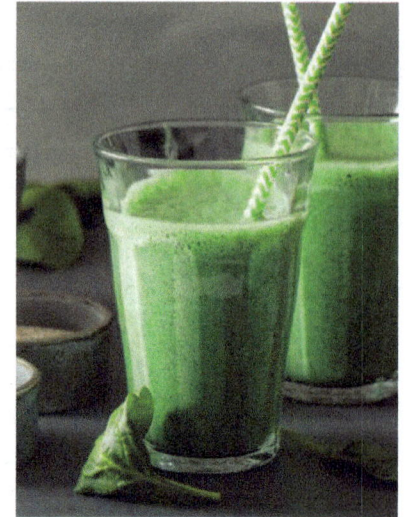

Nutritional Information (Per Serving)

- **Calories:** 170 kcal
- **Protein:** 4g
- **Carbohydrates:** 36g
- **Fiber:** 6g
- **Sugars:** 20g
- **Fats:** 3g
- **Saturated Fat:** 0.5g
- **Cholesterol:** 0mg
- **Sodium:** 40mg
- **Potassium:** 520mg

ANTI-INFLAMMATORY BLUEBERRY & KALE SMOOTHIE

Yield: 2 servings • Preparation Time: 5 minutes • Passive Time: None

Ingredients

> **1 cup** unsweetened almond milk (or oat milk for a thicker texture)
> **1 cup** frozen blueberries (high in antioxidants and anti-inflammatory compounds)
> **1 cup** fresh kale (a nutrient-dense leafy green rich in vitamins)
> **1/2** banana (for natural sweetness and potassium)
> **1 Tbsp** chia seeds (a source of omega-3 fatty acids and fiber)
> **1 tsp** ground flaxseed (adds fiber and omega-3s)
> **1/2 tsp** ground turmeric (optional, for additional anti-inflammatory benefits)
> **1/4 tsp** ground ginger (optional, for extra anti-inflammatory effects)
> **1 tsp** raw honey or maple syrup (optional, for added sweetness if desired)

Optional Add-ins:

> **1/4 cup** Greek yogurt or plant-based yogurt (for added creaminess and protein)
> **1 Tbsp** almond butter or walnut butter (for extra healthy fats and protein)

Instructions

1. **Prepare Ingredients**: Ensure the kale is rinsed and the banana is peeled and broken into chunks for easy blending.
2. **Combine in Blender**: Add the almond milk, blueberries, kale, banana, chia seeds, flaxseed, turmeric (if using), and ginger to the blender. Add yogurt or a nut butter if desired for added creaminess and nutritional benefits.
3. **Blend Until Smooth**: Blend on high until the mixture is smooth and creamy. If the smoothie is too thick, add a bit more almond milk to reach your desired consistency.
4. **Taste and Adjust**: Taste the smoothie, and if you prefer it a bit sweeter, add honey or maple syrup.
5. **Serve Immediately**: Pour the smoothie into two glasses. Add toppings if desired, and enjoy!

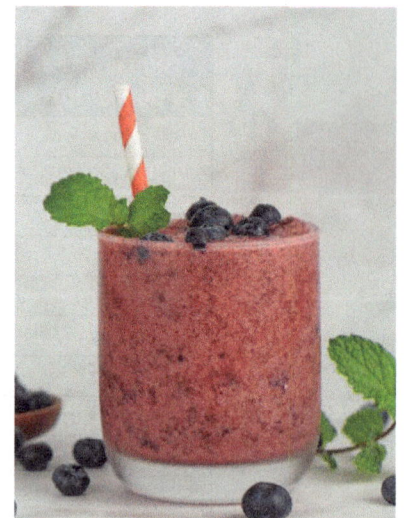

Nutritional Information (Per Serving)

- **Calories:** 180 kcal
- **Protein:** 4g
- **Carbohydrates:** 34g
- **Fiber:** 8g
- **Sugars:** 15g
- **Fats:** 4g
- **Saturated Fat:** 0.5g
- **Cholesterol:** 0mg
- **Sodium:** 40mg
- **Potassium:** 520mg

ORANGE & CARROT SUNRISE SMOOTHIE WITH TURMERIC

Yield: 2 servings • Preparation Time: 5 minutes • Passive Time: None

Ingredients

> **1 cup** fresh-squeezed orange juice (about 2 medium oranges)
> **1 cup** carrots, chopped (or **1/2 cup** carrot juice)
> **1/2 cup** frozen mango chunks (for creaminess and sweetness)
> **1/2 tsp** ground turmeric (or **1 inch** fresh turmeric root, peeled and grated)
> **1/2 tsp** grated ginger (optional, for extra warmth and anti-inflammatory properties)
> **1/2 cup** coconut water or filtered water (adjust for desired consistency)
> **1 tsp** lemon juice (optional, for added tang and vitamin C)

Optional Add-ins:

> **1 Tbsp** chia seeds (for added omega-3s and fiber)
> **1 Tbsp** Greek yogurt or coconut yogurt (for extra creaminess and probiotics)

Instructions

1. **Prepare Ingredients**: Juice the oranges if not using pre-squeezed juice, and chop the carrots if blending from fresh.
2. **Blend Ingredients**: Add the orange juice, carrots, frozen mango, turmeric, ginger, coconut water, and lemon juice (if using) to a high-speed blender. For a thicker texture, add Greek yogurt or chia seeds if desired.
3. **Blend Until Smooth**: Blend on high until the mixture is creamy and smooth. Adjust with a bit more coconut water if you prefer a thinner consistency.
4. **Taste and Adjust**: Taste the smoothie and add more ginger or lemon juice to suit your preference.
5. **Serve Immediately**: Pour into two glasses, add any desired toppings, and enjoy your nutrient-packed sunrise smoothie.

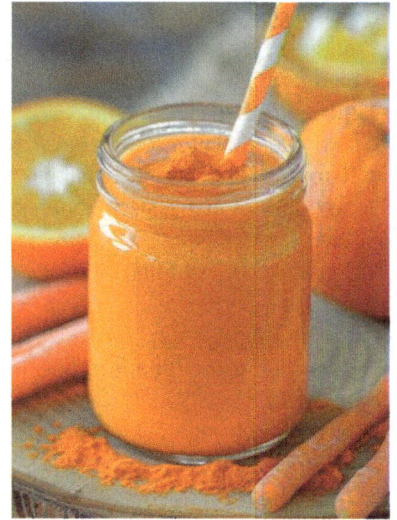

Nutritional Information (Per Serving)

- **Calories:** 120 kcal
- **Protein:** 2g
- **Carbohydrates:** 28g
- **Fiber:** 5g
- **Sugars:** 17g
- **Fats:** 0.5g
- **Saturated Fat:** 0g
- **Cholesterol:** 0mg
- **Sodium:** 30mg
- **Potassium:** 520mg

SPINACH & GREEN APPLE IMMUNITY BOOSTER

Yield: 2 servings • Preparation Time: 10 minutes • Passive Time: None

Ingredients

> **2 cups** fresh spinach leaves (washed)
> **1 medium** green apple, cored and chopped
> **1/2 inch** piece fresh ginger, peeled and grated (or **1/2 tsp** ground ginger)
> **1/2** cucumber, chopped (for hydration and a refreshing taste)
> **1 Tbsp** fresh lemon juice (from about 1/2 lemon)
> **1 cup** coconut water or filtered water (for hydration)
> **1 tsp** honey or maple syrup (optional, for added sweetness)

Optional Add-ins:

> **1/4 avocado** (for creaminess and healthy fats)
> **1 Tbsp** chia seeds or flaxseeds (for additional fiber and omega-3s)

Instructions

1. **Prepare Ingredients**: Wash the spinach leaves thoroughly. Core and chop the green apple, peel and grate the ginger, and chop the cucumber.
2. **Blend Ingredients**: In a blender, combine the spinach, green apple, ginger, cucumber, lemon juice, and coconut water. If using, add honey or maple syrup for sweetness and avocado for creaminess.
3. **Blend Until Smooth**: Blend on high speed until the mixture is smooth and creamy. If the mixture is too thick, add more coconut water or filtered water until you reach the desired consistency.
4. **Taste and Adjust**: Taste the booster and add more honey or lemon juice if you prefer a sweeter or tangier flavor.
5. **Serve Immediately**: Pour the smoothie into two glasses and enjoy your refreshing immunity booster right away.

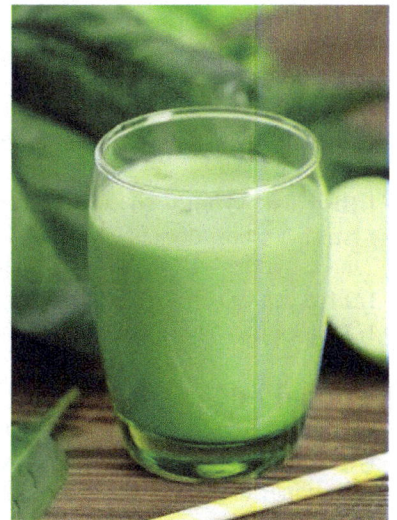

Nutritional Information (Per Serving)

- **Calories:** 90 kcal
- **Protein:** 2g
- **Carbohydrates:** 24g
- **Fiber:** 4g
- **Sugars:** 15g
- **Fats:** 1g
- **Saturated Fat:** 0g
- **Cholesterol:** 0mg
- **Sodium:** 35mg
- **Potassium:** 320mg

AVOCADO & KIWI ANTI-INFLAMMATORY SMOOTHIE

Yield: 2 servings • Preparation Time: 5 minutes • Passive Time: None

Ingredients
> **1 medium** ripe avocado, peeled and pitted
> **2 medium** ripe kiwis, peeled and chopped
> **1 cup** spinach leaves (fresh)
> **1 cup** coconut water (or filtered water)
> **1 Tbsp** fresh lime juice (from about 1 lime)
> **1 tsp** honey or maple syrup (optional, for added sweetness)
> **1/2 cup** ice cubes (optional, for a chilled smoothie)

Optional Add-ins:
> **1 Tbsp** chia seeds (for added fiber and omega-3s)
> **1/4 cup** Greek yogurt (for protein and creaminess)
> **1/2 tsp** ground turmeric (for extra anti-inflammatory benefits)

Instructions
1. **Prepare Ingredients**: Peel and pit the avocado and chop the kiwis. Wash the spinach leaves thoroughly.
2. **Blend Ingredients**: In a blender, combine the avocado, kiwis, spinach, coconut water, lime juice, and honey or maple syrup (if using). If desired, add chia seeds, Greek yogurt, and turmeric.
3. **Blend Until Smooth**: Blend on high speed until all ingredients are well combined and smooth. If you prefer a thicker consistency, you can add more avocado or yogurt.
4. **Adjust Consistency**: If the smoothie is too thick, add a bit more coconut water or water until you reach your desired consistency. If using ice, add it now and blend again until smooth.
5. **Serve Immediately**: Pour the smoothie into two glasses and enjoy!

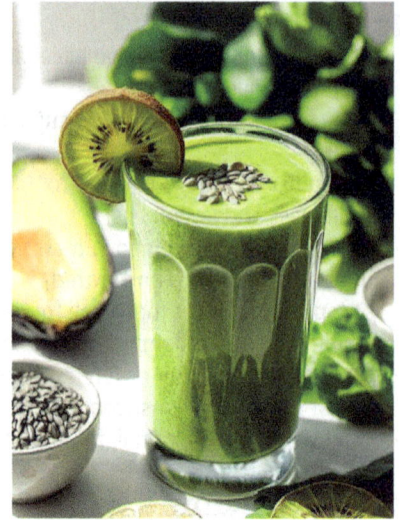

Nutritional Information (Per Serving)
- **Calories:** 190 kcal
- **Protein:** 4g
- **Carbohydrates:** 30g
- **Fiber:** 10g
- **Sugars:** 8g
- **Fats:** 9g
- **Saturated Fat:** 1g
- **Cholesterol:** 0mg
- **Sodium:** 25mg
- **Potassium:** 700mg

BLACKBERRY & BANANA OAT SMOOTHIE

Yield: 2 servings • Preparation Time: 5 minutes • Passive Time: None

Ingredients
> **1 cup** blackberries (fresh or frozen)
> **1 medium** ripe banana, peeled and sliced
> **1/2 cup** rolled oats (gluten-free if needed)
> **1 cup** almond milk (or any plant-based milk)
> **1 Tbsp** almond butter (or any nut butter)
> **1 tsp** chia seeds (optional, for added omega-3s)
> **1/2 tsp** vanilla extract
> **1/2 tsp** cinnamon (optional, for added flavor)

Optional Add-ins:
> **1 scoop** protein powder (for added protein)
> **1/2 cup** spinach (for added nutrients)
> **1 tsp** honey or maple syrup (for sweetness, if desired)

Instructions
1. **Prepare Ingredients**. If using fresh blackberries, rinse them under cold water. Peel and slice the banana. Gather all other ingredients.
2. **Blend Ingredients**: In a blender, combine the blackberries, banana, rolled oats, almond milk, almond butter, chia seeds (if using), vanilla extract, and cinnamon (if using).
3. **Blend Until Smooth**: Blend on high speed until the mixture is smooth and creamy. If the smoothie is too thick, you can add more almond milk to reach your desired consistency.
4. **Taste and Adjust**: Taste the smoothie and adjust sweetness by adding honey or maple syrup, if desired. Blend again briefly to mix.
5. **Serve Immediately**: Pour the smoothie into two glasses and enjoy!

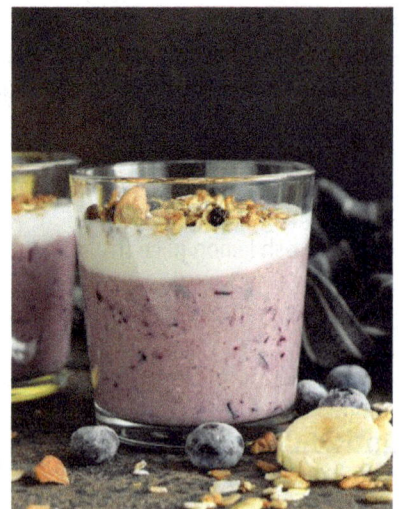

Nutritional Information (Per Serving)
- **Calories:** 290 kcal
- **Protein:** 7g
- **Carbohydrates:** 45g
- **Fiber:** 9g
- **Sugars:** 12g
- **Fats:** 10g
- **Saturated Fat:** 1g
- **Cholesterol:** 0mg
- **Sodium:** 150mg
- **Potassium:** 600mg

>

BOWLS & PORRIDGES

APPLE-CINNAMON OVERNIGHT OATS WITH WALNUTS

Yield: 2 servings • Preparation Time: 10 minutes • Passive Time: 4 hours (or overnight)

Ingredients
› **1 cup** rolled oats (gluten-free if needed)
› **1 1/2 cups** almond milk (or any plant-based milk)
› **1 medium** apple, diced (preferably a sweet variety like Fuji or Honeycrisp)
› **1 tsp** cinnamon
› **1/4 tsp** nutmeg (optional)
› **1 Tbsp** chia seeds (optional, for added omega-3s)
› **1 Tbsp** maple syrup or honey (optional, for sweetness)
› **1/4 cup** walnuts, chopped
› **1/2 tsp** vanilla extract

Optional Add-ins:
› **1 Tbsp** ground flaxseed (for additional fiber)
› **1/4 cup** raisins or dried cranberries (for extra sweetness and flavor)

Instructions
1. **Combine Dry Ingredients**: In a medium bowl, combine the rolled oats, chia seeds (if using), cinnamon, nutmeg (if using), and chopped walnuts.
2. **Mix Wet Ingredients**: In a separate bowl, whisk together the almond milk, maple syrup (or honey), and vanilla extract until well combined.
3. **Combine and Stir**: Pour the wet mixture over the dry ingredients and add the diced apple. Stir well to ensure all the oats are coated and the apple is evenly distributed.
4. **Transfer to Jars**: Divide the mixture into two jars or airtight containers. Make sure to leave some room at the top for the oats to expand as they absorb the liquid.
5. **Refrigerate**: Seal the containers and refrigerate for at least 4 hours or overnight. This allows the oats to soften and the flavors to meld.
6. **Serve**: When ready to eat, stir the oats. You can add a splash more almond milk if you prefer a thinner consistency. Top with additional chopped walnuts and fresh apple slices if desired.

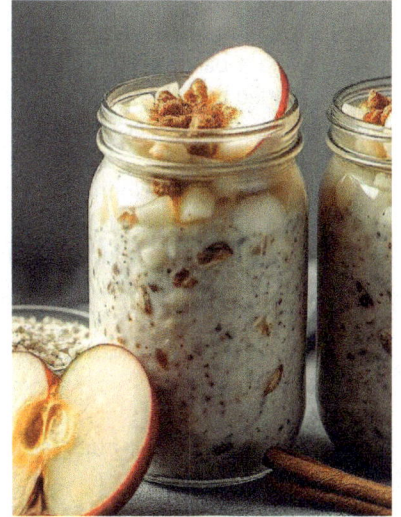

Nutritional Information (Per Serving)
- **Calories:** 325 kcal
- **Fats:** 10g
- **Protein:** 9g
- **Saturated Fat:** 1g
- **Carbohydrates:** 55g
- **Cholesterol:** 0mg
- **Fiber:** 9g
- **Sodium:** 160mg
- **Sugars:** 12g
- **Potassium:** 350mg

BUCKWHEAT & BERRY PORRIDGE WITH COCONUT MILK

Yield: 2 servings • Preparation Time: 5 minutes • Cooking Time: 15 minutes • Passive Time: None

Ingredients
› **1 cup** buckwheat groats
› **2 cups** water
› **1 cup** coconut milk (canned or carton)
› **1/2 cup** mixed berries (fresh or frozen; e.g., blueberries, raspberries, strawberries)
› **1 Tbsp** maple syrup or honey (optional, for sweetness)
› **1/2 tsp** cinnamon
› **1/4 tsp** vanilla extract
› **1 Tbsp** chia seeds (optional, for added fiber and omega-3s)
› **Pinch of salt**

Optional Toppings:
› Sliced banana or other fresh fruits
› Additional berries
› Chopped nuts (e.g., walnuts or almonds)
› Coconut flakes

Instructions
1. **Rinse the Buckwheat**: Place the buckwheat groats in a fine-mesh strainer and rinse under cold water to remove any bitterness. Drain well.
2. **Cook the Buckwheat**: In a medium saucepan, combine the rinsed buckwheat, water, and a pinch of salt. Bring to a boil over medium-high heat. Once boiling, reduce the heat to low, cover, and simmer for about 10-12 minutes, or until the buckwheat is tender and the water is absorbed.
3. **Add Coconut Milk and Berries**: Stir in the coconut milk, mixed berries, cinnamon, vanilla extract, and chia seeds (if using). Cook for an additional 2-3 minutes, stirring gently until the berries are warmed through and the porridge is creamy.
4. **Sweeten (Optional)**: Taste the porridge and add maple syrup or honey if you prefer it sweeter. Stir well to combine.
5. **Serve**: Divide the porridge into two bowls. Add your choice of toppings, such as additional berries, banana slices, chopped nuts, or coconut flakes.

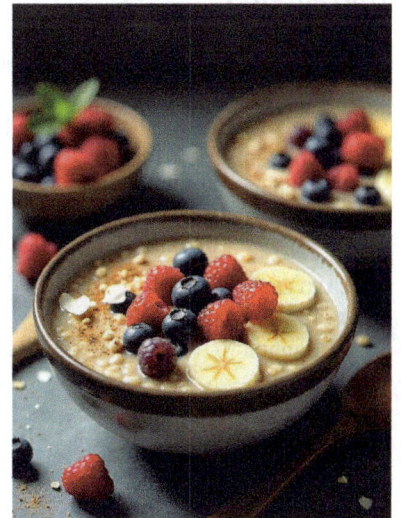

Nutritional Information (Per Serving)
- **Calories:** 340 kcal
- **Saturated Fat:** 9g
- **Protein:** 10g
- **Cholesterol:** 0mg
- **Carbohydrates:** 56g
- **Sodium:** 150mg
- **Fiber:** 9g
- **Potassium:** 400mg
- **Sugars:** 10g
- **Fats:** 12g

GOLDEN MILLET PORRIDGE WITH FIGS

Yield: 2 servings • Preparation Time: 5 minutes • Cooking Time: 20 minutes • Passive Time: None

Ingredients

> **1 cup** millet
> **3 cups** water or unsweetened almond milk (or any plant-based milk)
> **1/2 cup** dried figs, chopped
> **1/2 tsp** turmeric powder
> **1/2 tsp** cinnamon
> **1/4 tsp** ginger powder (optional, for extra anti-inflammatory benefits)
> **1 Tbsp** maple syrup or honey (optional, for sweetness)
> **Pinch of salt**
> **1 Tbsp** chia seeds (optional, for added fiber and omega-3s)

Optional Toppings:

> Sliced fresh figs or other fruits (e.g., bananas, berries)
> Chopped nuts (e.g., walnuts or almonds)
> A sprinkle of cinnamon
> Coconut flakes

Instructions

1. **Rinse the Millet**: Place the millet in a fine-mesh strainer and rinse under cold water to remove any debris. Drain well.
2. **Cook the Millet**: In a medium saucepan, combine the rinsed millet, water (or almond milk), turmeric, cinnamon, ginger (if using), and a pinch of salt. Bring to a boil over medium-high heat.
3. **Simmer**: Once boiling, reduce the heat to low, cover, and simmer for about 15 minutes, or until the millet is tender and the liquid is mostly absorbed. If using chia seeds, stir them in during the last 5 minutes of cooking.
4. **Add Figs and Sweeten**: Stir in the chopped dried figs and maple syrup (or honey) if using. Cook for an additional 2-3 minutes, allowing the figs to soften and the flavors to meld.
5. **Serve**: Divide the porridge into two bowls. Top with your choice of sliced fresh figs, nuts, or additional fruits.

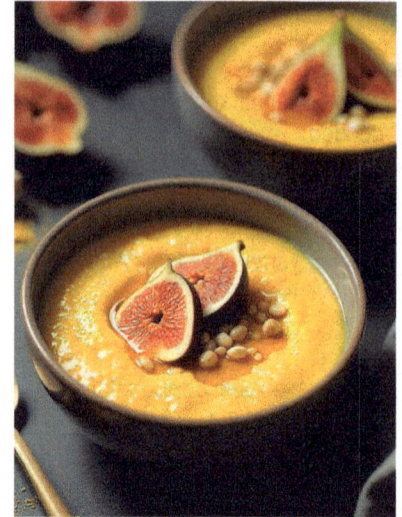

Nutritional Information (Per Serving)

- **Calories:** 325 kcal
- **Protein:** 9g
- **Carbohydrates:** 63g
- **Fiber:** 10g
- **Sugars:** 12g
- **Fats:** 6g
- **Saturated Fat:** 1g
- **Cholesterol:** 0mg
- **Sodium:** 150mg
- **Potassium:** 400mg

QUINOA BREAKFAST BOWL WITH CHERRIES AND HEMP SEEDS

Yield: 2 servings • Preparation Time: 10 minutes • Cooking Time: 15 minutes • Passive Time: None

Ingredients

> **1 cup** quinoa, rinsed
> **2 cups** water or unsweetened almond milk (or any plant-based milk)
> **1 cup** fresh or frozen cherries, pitted (if using frozen, thawed)
> **2 Tbsp** hemp seeds
> **1 Tbsp** chia seeds (optional, for added fiber)
> **1/2 tsp** cinnamon
> **1/4 tsp** vanilla extract (optional)
> **1 Tbsp** maple syrup or honey (optional, for sweetness)
> **Pinch of salt**

Optional Toppings:

> Additional fresh cherries or berries (blueberries, raspberries)
> Sliced banana
> Sliced almonds or walnuts
> Coconut flakes
> A dollop of almond or peanut butter

Instructions

1. **Rinse the Quinoa**: Place the quinoa in a fine-mesh strainer and rinse under cold running water for about 30 seconds. This helps to remove any bitterness from the quinoa.
2. **Cook the Quinoa**: In a medium saucepan, combine the rinsed quinoa, water (or almond milk), and a pinch of salt. Bring to a boil over medium-high heat.
3. **Simmer**: Once boiling, reduce the heat to low, cover, and let it simmer for about 15 minutes or until the quinoa is fluffy and the liquid is absorbed. Remove from heat and let it sit covered for an additional 5 minutes.
4. **Add Cherries and Flavor**: Fluff the quinoa with a fork and stir in the cherries, cinnamon, chia seeds (if using), vanilla extract (if using), and maple syrup (or honey) for sweetness.
5. **Serve**: Divide the quinoa mixture into two bowls. Top with hemp seeds and any additional toppings you prefer.

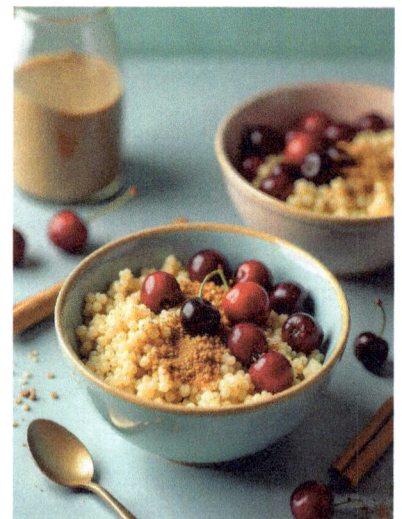

Nutritional Information (Per Serving)

- **Calories:** 310 kcal
- **Protein:** 10g
- **Carbohydrates:** 45g
- **Fiber:** 9g
- **Sugars:** 7g
- **Fats:** 9g
- **Saturated Fat:** 1g
- **Cholesterol:** 0mg
- **Sodium:** 130mg
- **Potassium:** 500mg

CHIA & HEMP SEED PUDDING WITH FRESH MANGO

Yield: 2 servings • Preparation Time: 10 minutes • Setting Time: 2 hours (or overnight)

Ingredients
> **1/4 cup** chia seeds
> **1/4 cup** hemp seeds
> **2 cups** almond milk (or any plant-based milk)
> **1 Tbsp** maple syrup or honey (optional, for sweetness)
> **1/2 tsp** vanilla extract (optional)
> **1/4 tsp** cinnamon (optional, for added flavor)
> **1 ripe** mango, diced (for topping)
> **Fresh mint leaves** (for garnish, optional)

Optional Toppings:
> Sliced almonds
> Additional hemp seeds
> Coconut flakes
> Berries (such as blueberries or strawberries)

Instructions
1. **Combine Ingredients**: In a medium-sized bowl or container, combine chia seeds, hemp seeds, almond milk, maple syrup (if using), vanilla extract, and cinnamon. Stir well to ensure all seeds are evenly distributed.
2. **Let It Set**: Cover the bowl/container and place it in the refrigerator. Allow the mixture to set for at least 2 hours, or overnight for the best texture. The chia seeds will absorb the liquid and thicken the mixture into a pudding-like consistency.
3. **Serve**: Once the pudding has set, give it a good stir to break up any clumps. Divide the pudding into two bowls or jars.
4. **Add Toppings**: Top each serving with diced mango and any optional toppings of your choice, such as sliced almonds, extra hemp seeds, coconut flakes, or berries. Garnish with fresh mint leaves if desired.

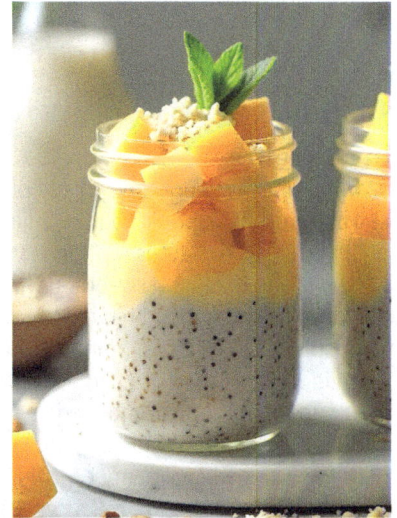

Nutritional Information (Per Serving)
- **Calories:** 320 kcal
- **Fats:** 18g
- **Protein:** 10g
- **Saturated Fat:** 1.5g
- **Carbohydrates:** 35g
- **Cholesterol:** 0mg
- **Fiber:** 12g
- **Sodium:** 150mg
- **Sugars:** 6g
- **Potassium:** 400mg

OATMEAL WITH TURMERIC, CINNAMON & APPLES

Yield: 2 servings • Preparation Time: 5 minutes • Cooking Time: 10 minutes

Ingredients
> **1 cup** rolled oats
> **2 cups** water or unsweetened almond milk
> **1 medium apple**, diced (preferably organic)
> **1/2 tsp** turmeric powder
> **1/2 tsp** cinnamon (or to taste)
> **1/4 tsp** salt
> **1 Tbsp** maple syrup or honey (optional for sweetness)
> **1 Tbsp** chia seeds (optional for added fiber and omega-3s)
> **1/4 cup** walnuts or pecans, chopped (for crunch and healthy fats)
> **1/2 tsp** vanilla extract (optional)

Instructions
1. **Prepare the Base**: In a medium saucepan, bring 2 cups of water (or almond milk) to a boil.
2. **Cook the Oats**: Once boiling, add 1 cup of rolled oats and salt. Reduce the heat to low, cover, and let simmer for about 5 minutes, stirring occasionally.
3. **Add Apples and Spices**: After 5 minutes, add the diced apple, turmeric, cinnamon, and chia seeds (if using). Stir well and continue to cook for an additional 3-5 minutes, or until the oats are tender and the apples are softened.
4. **Sweeten the Oatmeal**: Remove from heat and stir in maple syrup or honey (if desired) and vanilla extract.
5. **Serve**: Divide the oatmeal into bowls and top with chopped walnuts or pecans for added texture and flavor.

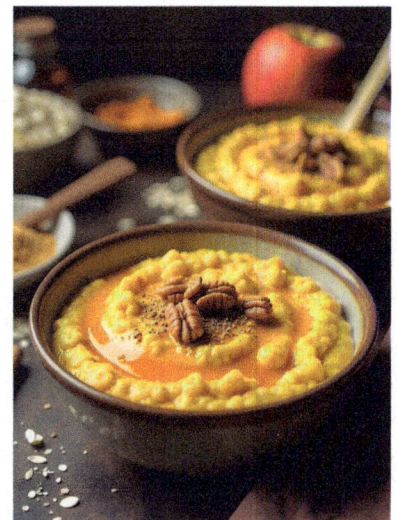

Nutritional Information (Per Serving)
- **Calories:** 350 kcal
- **Fats:** 12g
- **Protein:** 10g
- **Saturated Fat:** 1g
- **Carbohydrates:** 58g
- **Cholesterol:** 0mg
- **Fiber:** 9g
- **Sodium:** 150mg
- **Sugars:** 8g
- **Potassium:** 500mg

>

2. SNACKS AND APPETIZERS
DIPS & SPREADS

AVOCADO-LIME GUACAMOLE WITH FRESH CILANTRO

Yield: 4 servings • Preparation Time: 10 minutes • Total Time: 10 minutes

Ingredients
> **2 large** ripe avocados, peeled and pitted
> **1 Tbsp** fresh lime juice (about 1/2 lime)
> **1/2 cup** diced tomatoes (optional: grape or cherry tomatoes for a sweeter flavor)
> **1/4 cup** finely chopped red onion
> **1 Tbsp** minced jalapeño (remove seeds for a milder flavor)
> **1/4 cup** fresh cilantro, chopped
> **1/4 tsp** sea salt (or to taste)
> **1/8 tsp** ground black pepper

Optional Add-ins for Extra Flavor
> **1 clove** garlic, minced
> **1 Tbsp** hemp seeds (for added omega-3s and protein)
> **1 Tbsp** extra-virgin olive oil (adds healthy fats)

Instructions
1. **Prepare Avocado Base**: In a medium mixing bowl, scoop out the avocado flesh and mash it gently with a fork, leaving some chunks for texture.
2. **Add Lime Juice**: Immediately add lime juice to the avocado to prevent browning and enhance flavor. Stir to combine.
3. **Incorporate Vegetables**: Add diced tomatoes, red onion, and jalapeño. Stir gently to evenly distribute.
4. **Season with Herbs & Spices**: Add the chopped cilantro, salt, and black pepper. If using, mix in minced garlic, hemp seeds, or a drizzle of olive oil for added benefits.
5. **Taste and Adjust**: Adjust seasoning to your taste, adding more lime juice, salt, or pepper if desired.
6. **Serve Immediately**: For optimal flavor and texture, serve the guacamole immediately. If not serving right away, cover tightly with plastic wrap, pressing it against the surface of the guacamole to prevent oxidation.

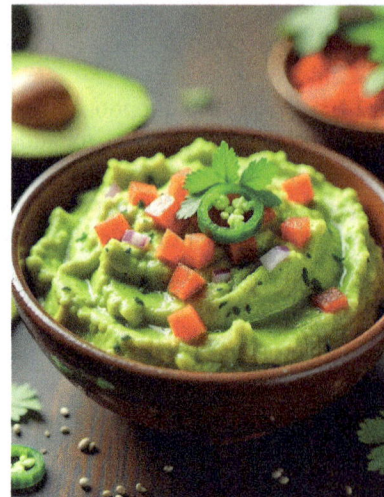

Nutritional Information (Per Serving)
- **Calories:** 130 kcal
- **Protein:** 2g
- **Carbohydrates:** 8g
- **Fiber:** 5g
- **Sugars:** 1g
- **Fats:** 11g
- **Saturated Fat:** 1.5g
- **Cholesterol:** 0mg
- **Sodium:** 150mg
- **Potassium:** 485mg

ARTICHOKE & SPINACH HUMMUS WITH TAHINI

Yield: 6 servings • Preparation Time: 10 minutes • Passive Time: 10 minutes (if draining canned artichokes)

Ingredients
> **1 1/2 cups** canned or cooked artichoke hearts, drained and rinsed
> **1 cup** fresh spinach, lightly packed
> **1 cup** cooked chickpeas, rinsed and drained
> **3 Tbsp** tahini
> **2 Tbsp** extra-virgin olive oil
> **2 Tbsp** lemon juice (about half a lemon)
> **1 clove** garlic, minced
> **1/2 tsp** ground turmeric
> **1/4 tsp** ground cumin
> **1/4 tsp** sea salt (or to taste)
> **1/8 tsp** black pepper
> **2–3 Tbsp** water (to adjust consistency)

Optional Ingredients for Added Flavor or Nutrition
> **1/4 tsp** smoked paprika (adds depth)
> **1 Tbsp** nutritional yeast (adds a cheesy flavor)
> **1/8 tsp** cayenne pepper (for a hint of spice)

Instructions
1. **Prepare Ingredients:** Drain and rinse the artichoke hearts and chickpeas. Measure out the spinach, olive oil, tahini, lemon juice, garlic, and spices.
2. **Blend the Ingredients:** In a food processor or high-speed blender, combine the artichokes, spinach, chickpeas, tahini, olive oil, lemon juice, garlic, turmeric, cumin, salt, and black pepper. Blend until smooth, pausing to scrape down the sides as needed.
3. **Adjust Consistency:** Add water, 1 Tbsp at a time, to reach your preferred consistency. Blend until creamy and smooth.
4. **Taste and Adjust Seasoning:** Taste the hummus and adjust salt, pepper, or lemon juice if desired. Add any optional ingredients, like smoked paprika or cayenne, for additional flavor.
5. **Serve:** Transfer to a bowl and top with a drizzle of olive oil, a sprinkle of turmeric or paprika, and a few extra artichoke or chickpea pieces if desired.

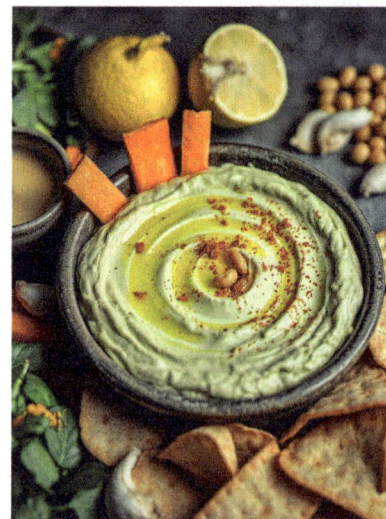

Nutritional Information (per serving)
- **Calories:** 145 kcal
- **Protein:** 4 g
- **Carbohydrates:** 11 g
- **Fats:** 9 g
- **Fiber:** 4 g
- **Cholesterol:** 0 mg
- **Sodium:** 140 mg
- **Potassium:** 225 mg

TURMERIC-SPICED YOGURT DIP WITH DILL

Yield: 4 servings • Preparation Time: 5 minutes • Passive Time: 5–10 minutes (to allow flavors to meld)

Ingredients

> **1 cup** Greek yogurt (unsweetened, plain)
> **1 Tbsp** fresh dill, finely chopped
> **1/2 tsp** ground turmeric
> **1/4 tsp** ground cumin
> **1 clove** garlic, minced
> **1 Tbsp** lemon juice (about half a lemon)
> **1/4 tsp** sea salt (or to taste)
> **1/8 tsp** black pepper
> **1–2 Tbsp** water (to adjust consistency)

Optional Ingredients for Added Flavor or Nutrition

> **1/4 tsp** smoked paprika (for additional depth of flavor)
> **1 Tbsp** olive oil (for a richer taste and added healthy fats)
> **1/4 tsp** cayenne pepper (for a touch of heat)

Instructions

1. **Prepare the Ingredients**: Measure out the Greek yogurt and finely chop the dill. Mince the garlic.
2. **Combine Ingredients:** In a medium bowl, mix together the yogurt, dill, turmeric, cumin, garlic, lemon juice, salt, and black pepper.
3. **Adjust Consistency:** Add 1–2 Tbsp of water if you prefer a thinner dip. Stir until smooth and well combined.
4. **Taste and Adjust Seasoning:** Taste the dip and adjust salt, pepper, or lemon juice as needed. Add any optional ingredients, like smoked paprika or olive oil, for extra flavor.
5. **Let It Rest**: Allow the dip to sit for 5–10 minutes for the flavors to meld. This resting time enhances the anti-inflammatory benefits by allowing the turmeric to blend with the yogurt's fat content.
6. **Serve:** Transfer to a serving dish, drizzle with olive oil if desired, and garnish with a sprinkle of fresh dill or paprika.

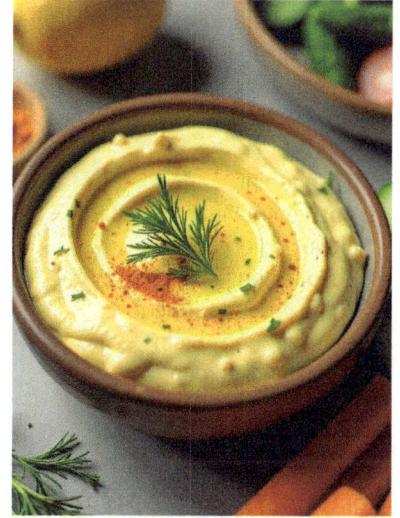

Nutritional Information (per serving)

- **Calories**: 80 kcal
- **Protein**: 5 g
- **Carbohydrates**: 5 g
- **Fats**: 4 g
- **Fiber**: 0 g
- **Cholesterol**: 7 mg
- **Sodium**: 180 mg
- **Potassium**: 170 mg

CILANTRO & LIME WHITE BEAN DIP

Yield: 4 servings • Preparation Time: 10 minutes • Cooking Time: None (just blend and serve!)

Ingredients

> **1 can** (15 oz) cannellini or white beans, rinsed and drained
> **2 Tbsp** extra-virgin olive oil
> **2 Tbsp** lime juice (about 1 lime)
> **1 clove** garlic, minced
> **1/4 tsp** sea salt (or to taste)
> **1/4 tsp** ground cumin
> **1/8 tsp** black pepper
> **1/4 cup** fresh cilantro leaves, chopped

Optional Ingredients for Extra Flavor or Nutrition

> **1/4 tsp** cayenne pepper (for heat)
> **1 Tbsp** tahini (for creaminess and a nutty flavor)
> **1 tsp** lime zest (for added citrus notes)
> **2 Tbsp** chopped green onions (for garnish)

Instructions

1. **Prepare Ingredients**: Rinse and drain the beans thoroughly. Chop the cilantro and mince the garlic.
2. **Blend the Dip:** In a food processor, combine the white beans, olive oil, lime juice, garlic, salt, cumin, black pepper, and cilantro. Blend until smooth, stopping to scrape down the sides as needed. If you prefer a thinner consistency, add a splash of water and blend again.
3. **Adjust Seasoning:** Taste and adjust seasoning. Add more lime juice for extra brightness, or increase the salt and pepper as desired. If you like a bit of spice, mix in the optional cayenne pepper.
4. **Serve and Garnish:** Transfer to a serving bowl. Optionally, top with a drizzle of olive oil, extra chopped cilantro, green onions, or a sprinkle of lime zest for added flavor and visual appeal.

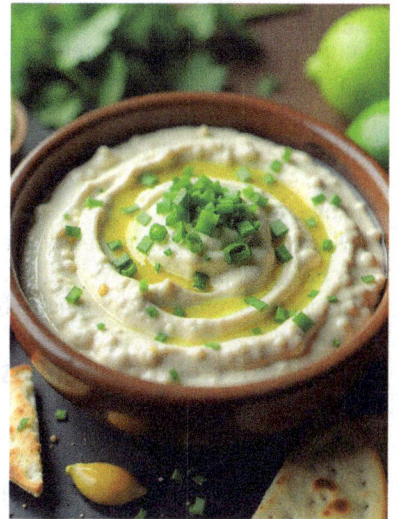

Nutritional Information (per serving)

- **Calories**: 135 kcal
- **Protein**: 4 g
- **Carbohydrates**: 16 g
- **Fats**: 6 g
- **Fiber**: 4 g
- **Cholesterol**: 0 mg
- **Sodium**: 210 mg
- **Potassium**: 300 mg

TURMERIC PUMPKIN HUMMUS

Yield: 4 servings • Preparation Time: 10 minutes • Cooking Time: 5 minutes (optional if using canned pumpkin)

Ingredients

> **1 cup** canned pumpkin puree (or freshly cooked pumpkin)
> **1 can (15 oz)** chickpeas, drained and rinsed
> **2 Tbsp** tahini
> **2 Tbsp** extra-virgin olive oil
> **1 clove** garlic, minced
> **1 Tbsp** lemon juice
> **1/2 tsp** ground turmeric
> **1/2 tsp** ground cumin
> **1/4 tsp** smoked paprika
> **1/4 tsp** ground black pepper
> **1/4 tsp** sea salt, or to taste
> **2–4 Tbsp** water (to adjust consistency)

Optional Ingredients for Extra Flavor or Nutrition

> **1/4 tsp** cayenne pepper (for a spicy kick)
> **1 tsp** grated fresh ginger (for added anti-inflammatory benefits)
> **1/2 tsp** ground cinnamon (for warmth and added anti-inflammatory properties)

Instructions

1. **Prepare the Base Ingredients:** In a food processor, combine the pumpkin puree, chickpeas, tahini, olive oil, minced garlic, and lemon juice.
2. **Add Spices:** Add turmeric, cumin, smoked paprika, black pepper, and sea salt to the food processor. If using, add cayenne pepper, fresh ginger, or cinnamon.
3. **Blend Until Smooth:** Process the mixture until it's smooth and creamy, pausing to scrape down the sides as needed. Gradually add water (1 Tbsp at a time) until you reach your desired consistency.
4. **Taste and Adjust:** Taste the hummus and adjust seasonings if needed. Add more lemon juice for acidity or a pinch more salt as desired.
5. **Serve:** Transfer to a serving bowl and garnish with a drizzle of olive oil, a sprinkle of smoked paprika, or extra turmeric for color.

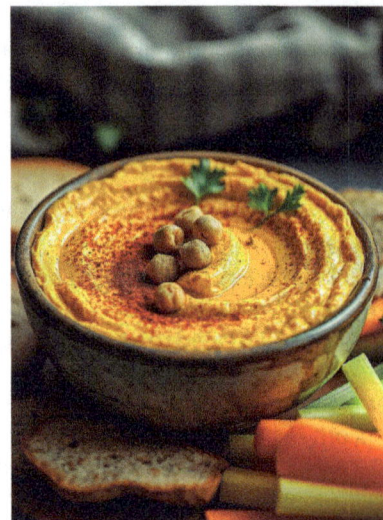

Nutritional Information (per serving)

- **Calories**: 180 kcal
- **Protein**: 5 g
- **Carbohydrates**: 17 g
- **Fats**: 10 g
- **Fiber**: 5 g
- **Cholesterol**: 0 mg
- **Sodium**: 240 mg
- **Potassium**: 300 mg

GREEN OLIVE & BASIL ANTI-INFLAMMATORY TAPENADE

Yield: 4 servings • Preparation Time: 10 minutes • Cooking Time: No cooking required

Ingredients

> **1 cup** green olives, pitted (preferably Kalamata or Castelvetrano)
> **1/4 cup** fresh basil leaves, packed
> **2 Tbsp** extra-virgin olive oil
> **1 Tbsp** capers, rinsed
> **1 clove** garlic, minced
> **1/2 tsp** lemon juice (or more to taste)
> **1/4 tsp** black pepper
> **1/4 tsp** red pepper flakes (optional for a spicy kick)

Optional Ingredients for Extra Flavor or Nutrition

> **1 Tbsp** nutritional yeast (for a cheesy flavor and added B vitamins)
> **1/4 cup** chopped walnuts or almonds (for added crunch and omega-3 fatty acids)

Instructions

1. **Prepare Ingredients:**
   Gather all ingredients, rinsing and draining the capers if necessary. If using walnuts or almonds, chop them roughly.
2. **Combine Ingredients:** In a food processor, combine the green olives, basil leaves, olive oil, capers, minced garlic, lemon juice, black pepper, and red pepper flakes (if using).
3. **Blend Until Smooth:** Pulse the mixture until it reaches your desired consistency. For a chunkier tapenade, pulse briefly; for a smoother texture, blend longer.
4. **Taste and Adjust:** Taste the tapenade and adjust the lemon juice, salt, or pepper according to your preferences.
5. **Optional Step:** If using, fold in the chopped nuts or sprinkle nutritional yeast for added flavor and nutrition.
6. **Serve:** Transfer the tapenade to a serving bowl. Drizzle with additional olive oil if desired.

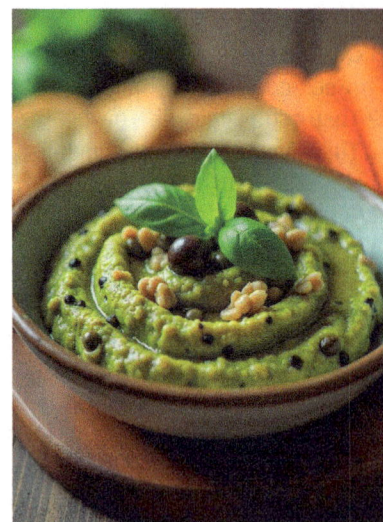

Nutritional Information (per serving)

- **Calories**: 90 kcal
- **Protein**: 1 g
- **Carbohydrates**: 3 g
- **Fats**: 9 g
- **Fiber**: 1 g
- **Cholesterol**: 0 mg
- **Sodium**: 300 mg (varies based on olive and caper brand)
- **Potassium**: 150 mg

>

CAULIFLOWER TOTS WITH CURRY

Yield: 4 servings • Preparation Time: 15 minutes • Cooking Time: 25 minutes

Ingredients

> 1 **medium** head of cauliflower
> **1/2 cup** almond flour
> **1/4 cup** nutritional yeast
> **1/4 tsp** turmeric powder (for its anti-inflammatory properties)
> **1/2 tsp** curry powder)
> **1/2 tsp** garlic powder
> **1/4 tsp** onion powder
> **1/4 tsp** black pepper
> **1/2 tsp** sea salt (adjust to taste)
> **1 large** egg (or flax egg for a vegan option)
> **1 Tbsp** olive oil (for greasing the baking sheet)

Optional Ingredients for Extra Flavor or Nutrition

> **1/4 tsp** cayenne pepper (for heat)
> **1/4 cup** grated carrot (for added nutrition and color)

Instructions

1. **Preheat the Oven:** Heat to 400°F (200°C) and prepare a greased, parchment-lined baking sheet.
2. **Rice the Cauliflower:** Remove the leaves and stem from the cauliflower and cut it into florets. You can also grate it with a box grater if a food processor is not available.
3. **Cook the Cauliflower:** Transfer the riced cauliflower to a microwave-safe bowl and microwave on high for 4–5 minutes, or until softened. Allow it to cool slightly.
4. **Mix the Ingredients:** In a large bowl, combine the riced cauliflower, almond flour, nutritional yeast, turmeric, curry powder, garlic powder, onion powder, black pepper, sea salt, and grated carrot (if using). Stir until well mixed.
5. **Add the Egg:** Beat the egg in a small bowl and add it to the cauliflower mixture. Stir until everything is well combined. The mixture should hold together.
6. **Form the Tots:** Using your hands, form small tot shapes (about 1 inch long) and place them on the prepared baking sheet.
7. **Bake:** Bake the cauliflower tots in the preheated oven for 20–25 minutes, or until they are golden brown and crispy. Flip them halfway through cooking to ensure even browning.
8. **Serve:** Remove the tots from the oven and let them cool for a couple of minutes. Serve warm, garnished with fresh cilantro or parsley if desired.

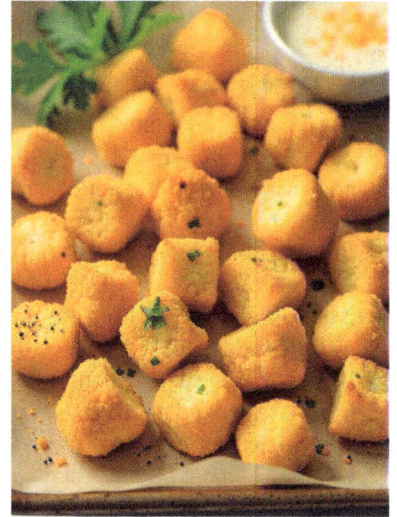

Nutritional Information (per serving)

- **Calories**: 130 kcal
- **Protein**: 5 g
- **Carbohydrates**: 8 g
- **Fats**: 9 g
- **Fiber**: 3 g
- **Cholesterol**: 40 mg
- **Sodium**: 300 mg
- **Potassium**: 230 mg

SPICED LENTIL FRITTERS WITH MINT YOGURT SAUCE

Yield: 4 servings • Preparation Time: 15 minutes • Cooking Time: 25 minutes

Ingredients
For the Fritters:

> **1 cup** cooked lentils (green or brown)
> **1/2 cup** grated carrot
> **1/4 cup** finely chopped onion
> **1/4 cup** chopped fresh cilantro
> **2 cloves** garlic, minced
> **1/2 tsp** ground cumin
> **1/2 tsp** ground coriander
> **1/4 tsp** turmeric powder
> **1/4 tsp** cayenne pepper (optional)
> **1/2 tsp** sea salt (adjust to taste)
> **1/2 cup** almond flour (or whole wheat flour)
> **1 egg**, beaten (or flax egg for vegan option)

For the Mint Yogurt Sauce:

> **1 cup** plain yogurt (Greek yogurt for added protein)
> **1/4 cup** fresh mint leaves, chopped
> **1 tsp** lemon juice
> **1/2 tsp** sea salt (adjust to taste)
> **1/4 tsp** black pepper

Optional Ingredients

> **1/4 tsp** smoked paprika (for extra flavor)
> **Chopped green onions** for garnish

Instructions

1. **Prepare the Fritter Mixture:** In a large bowl, combine cooked lentils, grated carrot, chopped onion, cilantro, minced garlic, cumin, coriander, turmeric, cayenne pepper, sea salt, almond flour, and beaten egg. Mix until well combined.
2. **Form the Fritters:** Using your hands, shape the mixture into small patties (about 2 inches in diameter).
3. **Cook the Fritters:** Heat a non-stick skillet and add a drizzle of olive oil. Once hot, add the fritters in batches, cooking on each side or until golden brown and crispy. Remove from the skillet and set aside.
4. **Prepare the Mint Yogurt Sauce:** In a separate bowl, mix together yogurt, chopped mint, lemon juice, salt, and black pepper until well blended.
5. **Serve the Fritters:** Arrange the fritters on a serving plate and drizzle with the mint yogurt sauce. Garnish with chopped green onions, if desired.

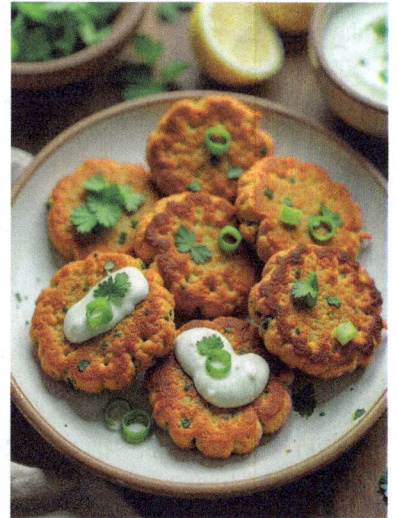

Nutritional Information (per serving)

- **Calories**: 170 kcal
- **Protein**: 8 g
- **Carbohydrates**: 24 g
- **Fats**: 5 g
- **Fiber**: 6 g
- **Cholesterol**: 30 mg
- **Sodium**: 220 mg
- **Potassium**: 300 mg

SWEET POTATO AVOCADO TOAST WITH MICROGREENS

Yield: 2 servings • Preparation Time: 10 minutes • Cooking Time: 20 minutes

Ingredients

› **1 medium** sweet potato (about 8 oz)
› **1 ripe** avocado
› **1/2 cup** microgreens (such as arugula, broccoli, or radish)
› **2 slices** whole grain bread (preferably sprouted for added nutrients)
› **1 Tbsp** olive oil (plus extra for drizzling)
› **1/2 tsp** sea salt (adjust to taste)
› **1/4 tsp** black pepper
› **1/4 tsp** garlic powder (optional)
› **1/4 tsp** crushed red pepper flakes (optional, for heat)
› **Juice of 1/2 lime** (optional, for added flavor)

Optional Ingredients for Extra Taste or Nutrition

› **1 Tbsp** hemp seeds (for added protein and omega-3 fatty acids)
› **1 Tbsp** chopped fresh cilantro or parsley (for garnish)
› **1/4 tsp** smoked paprika (for a smoky flavor)

Instructions

1. **Preheat the Oven:** Preheat your oven to 400°F (200°C).
2. **Prepare the Sweet Potato:** Peel and cut the sweet potato into 1/2-inch cubes. Toss the cubes in a bowl with olive oil, sea salt, black pepper, garlic powder, and optional smoked paprika. Spread them in a single layer on a baking sheet lined with parchment paper.
3. **Roast the Sweet Potato:** Roast the sweet potato in the preheated oven for 20 minutes, or until fork-tender, tossing halfway through for even cooking.
4. **Toast the Bread:** While the sweet potatoes are roasting, toast your whole grain bread slices until crispy.
5. **Mash the Avocado:** In a bowl, scoop the ripe avocado and mash it with a fork. Add lime juice, if using, and season with a pinch of salt and pepper.
6. **Assemble the Toast:** Once the sweet potatoes are done, remove them from the oven. Spread a generous layer of mashed avocado on each slice of toast.
7. **Top with Sweet Potatoes and Microgreens:** Arrange the roasted sweet potato cubes on top of the avocado spread, followed by a handful of microgreens. Drizzle with a little olive oil and sprinkle with crushed red pepper flakes, if desired.

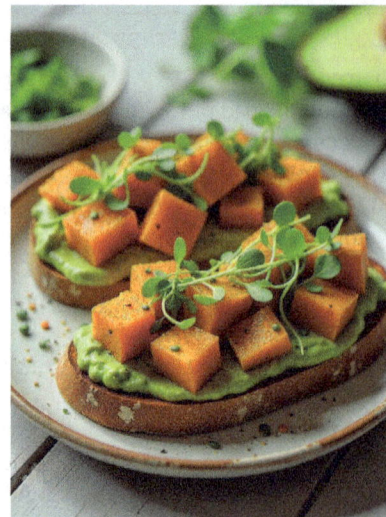

Nutritional Information (per serving)

- **Calories**: 320 kcal
- **Protein**: 7 g
- **Carbohydrates**: 40 g
- **Fats**: 16 g
- **Fiber**: 10 g
- **Cholesterol**: 0 mg
- **Sodium**: 300 mg
- **Potassium**: 800 mg

AVOCADO-STUFFED MUSHROOMS WITH GARLIC

Yield: 4 servings (8 stuffed mushrooms) • Preparation Time: 10 minutes • Cooking Time: 15 minutes

Ingredients

› **8 large** portobello mushrooms or baby bella mushrooms
› **1 ripe** avocado, mashed
› **2 cloves** garlic, minced
› **1 tbsp** olive oil
› **1 tbsp** lemon juice (freshly squeezed)
› **1/4 tsp** sea salt
› **1/4 tsp** black pepper
› **1/4 tsp** smoked paprika (optional for added flavor)
› **2 tbsp** fresh parsley, chopped (for garnish)
› **1/4 cup** cherry tomatoes, diced (optional for topping)

Optional Ingredients

› **1/4 tsp** red pepper flakes (for a bit of heat)
› **2 tbsp** nutritional yeast (for a cheesy flavor)

Instructions

1. **Preheat the Oven:** Preheat your oven to 375°F (190°C).
2. **Prepare the Mushrooms:** Clean the mushrooms by gently wiping them with a damp cloth. Remove the stems and carefully scoop out the gills if using portobello mushrooms to create more space for the filling.
3. **Make the Avocado Filling:** In a bowl, mash the ripe avocado with a fork. Add minced garlic, olive oil, lemon juice, sea salt, black pepper, and smoked paprika (if using). Mix until well combined.
4. **Stuff the Mushrooms:** Fill each mushroom cap generously with the avocado mixture, using a spoon to pack it in gently.
5. **Bake the Stuffed Mushrooms:** Arrange the stuffed mushrooms on a baking sheet lined with parchment paper. Bake in the preheated oven for 15 minutes, or until the mushrooms are tender and the tops are slightly golden.
6. **Garnish and Serve:** Remove from the oven and let cool slightly. Garnish with chopped parsley and diced cherry tomatoes (if using) before serving.

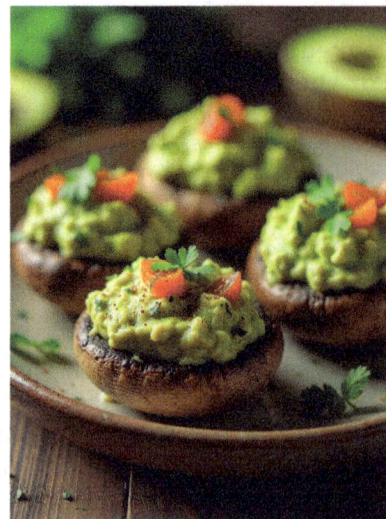

Nutritional Information (per serving, 2 stuffed mushrooms)

- **Calories**: 150 kcal
- **Protein**: 3 g
- **Carbohydrates**: 10 g
- **Fats**: 12 g
- **Fiber**: 5 g
- **Cholesterol**: 0 mg
- **Sodium**: 250 mg
- **Potassium**: 450 mg

ZUCCHINI & CHICKPEA BITES WITH TAHINI DIP

Yield: 4 servings (approximately 12 bites) • Preparation Time: 15 minutes • Cooking Time: 20 minutes

Ingredients
For the Zucchini & Chickpea Bites:
› **1 medium** zucchini, grated (about 1 cup)
› **1 cup** canned chickpeas, drained and rinsed
› **1/4 cup** almond flour (or more as needed)
› **1/4 cup** finely chopped onion
› **2 cloves** garlic, minced
› **1/2 tsp** ground cumin
› **1/2 tsp** smoked paprika
› **1/4 tsp** sea salt
› **1/4 tsp** black pepper
› **1 tbsp** fresh parsley or cilantro, chopped (optional)

For the Tahini Dip:
› **1/4 cup** tahini
› **2 tbsp** lemon juice (freshly squeezed)
› **1 clove** garlic, minced
› **1-2 tbsp** water (to thin the dip)
› **Salt and pepper** to taste

Optional Ingredients
› **1/4 tsp** cayenne pepper (for heat)
› **1 tbsp** nutritional yeast (for added flavor and nutrients)

Instructions
1. **Preheat the Oven:** Preheat your oven to 375°F (190°C) and line a baking sheet with parchment paper.
2. **Prepare the Zucchini:** Grate the zucchini and place it in a clean kitchen towel. Squeeze out excess moisture to ensure the bites hold together well.
3. **Combine the Ingredients:** In a mixing bowl, mash the chickpeas with a fork until mostly smooth. Add the grated zucchini, almond flour, chopped onion, minced garlic, cumin, smoked paprika, sea salt, black pepper, and optional parsley or cilantro. Mix until well combined. If the mixture is too wet, add a bit more almond flour.
4. **Shape the Bites:** Using your hands, form the mixture into small balls or patties, about 1-2 inches in diameter. Place them on the prepared baking sheet.
5. **Bake the Bites:** Bake in the preheated oven for 20 minutes, flipping halfway through, until golden brown and firm.
6. **Make the Tahini Dip:** While the bites are baking, whisk together the tahini, lemon juice, minced garlic, and water in a small bowl. Adjust the consistency with more water if needed, and season with salt and pepper to taste.
7. **Serve and Enjoy:** Once the bites are done, remove them from the oven and let them cool slightly. Serve warm with the tahini dip on the side.

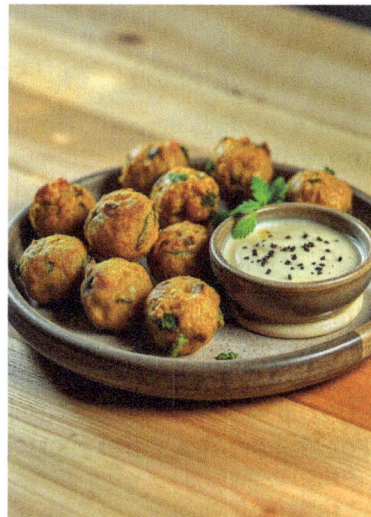

Nutritional Information (per serving, 3 bites with dip)
- **Calories**: 180 kcal
- **Protein**: 6 g
- **Carbohydrates**: 20 g
- **Fats**: 9 g
- **Fiber**: 6 g
- **Cholesterol**: 0 mg
- **Sodium**: 250 mg
- **Potassium**: 450 mg

KALE & SWEET POTATO MINI TARTS

Yield: 12 mini tarts • Preparation Time: 20 minutes • Cooking Time: 30 minutes (plus cooling time)

Ingredients
› **1 medium** sweet potato (about 1 cup, peeled and grated)
› **1 cup** kale, finely chopped (stems removed)
› **1/2 cup** almond flour
› **1/4 cup** coconut flour
› **2 tbsp** olive oil
› **2 tbsp** nutritional yeast (optional, for a cheesy flavor)
› **1 clove** garlic, minced
› **1/2 tsp** ground turmeric
› **1/4 tsp** black pepper
› **1/2 tsp** sea salt
› **1/4 tsp** cayenne pepper (optional, for heat)
› **1 egg** (or flax egg for a vegan option)
› **1/4 cup** water (or as needed)

Optional Toppings
› Sliced avocado
› **Chopped fresh herbs** (parsley or cilantro)
› **Crumbled feta cheese** (for added creaminess)

Instructions
1. **Preheat the Oven:** Preheat your oven to 375°F (190°C).
2. **Prepare the Sweet Potato:** Peel and grate the sweet potato using a box grater or food processor. Place it in a large bowl.
3. **Sauté the Kale:** In a small skillet, heat 1 tbsp of olive oil over medium heat. Add minced garlic and sauté for about 1 minute until fragrant. Add the chopped kale and cook for an additional 3-4 minutes until wilted. Remove from heat and add to the bowl with grated sweet potato.
4. **Make the Tart Crust:** In the bowl with sweet potato and kale, add almond flour, coconut flour, nutritional yeast, turmeric, black pepper, sea salt, cayenne pepper (if using), and the egg. Mix until well combined, then gradually add water as needed to form a dough that holds together but isn't sticky.
5. **Form the Mini Tarts:** Grease a muffin tin with the remaining 1 tbsp of olive oil. Scoop about 1-2 tbsp of the dough into each muffin cup and press it down to form a crust. Use your fingers to shape the crust, making sure to cover the sides well.
6. **Bake the Tarts:** Place the muffin tin in the preheated oven and bake for 20-25 minutes, or until the edges are golden brown. Remove from the oven and let cool for about 10 minutes before carefully removing the tarts from the tin.
7. **Fill the Tarts:** Once cooled slightly, you can fill each tart with any additional toppings such as sliced avocado, chopped herbs, or crumbled feta cheese.

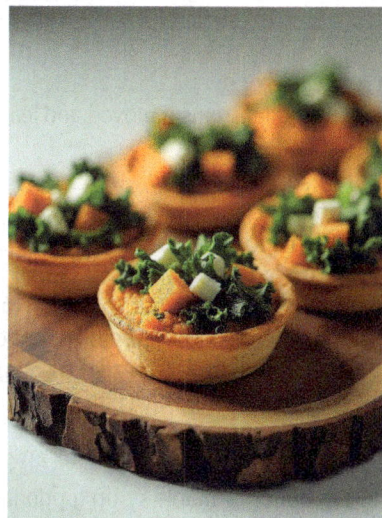

Nutritional Information (per mini tart)
- **Calories**: 120 kcal
- **Protein**: 3 g
- **Carbohydrates**: 10 g
- **Fats**: 8 g
- **Fiber**: 2 g
- **Cholesterol**: 30 mg (if using egg)
- **Sodium**: 150 mg
- **Potassium**: 250 mg

3. SALAD RECIPES
LEAFY GREEN SALADS

ARUGULA, APPLE & PECAN SALAD WITH LEMON VINAIGRETTE

Yield: 4 servings • Preparation Time: 10 minutes • Cooking Time: None

Ingredients

> **4 cups** fresh arugula, washed and dried
> **1 medium** apple (such as Fuji or Honeycrisp), cored and thinly sliced
> **1/2 cup** pecans, roughly chopped (toasted for extra flavor)
> **1/4 cup** crumbled goat cheese or feta (optional)
> **1/4 cup** red onion, thinly sliced (optional)

For the Lemon Vinaigrette:

> **3 tbsp** extra virgin olive oil
> **2 tbsp** fresh lemon juice
> **1 tsp** Dijon mustard
> **1 tsp** honey or maple syrup (optional)
> **Salt and black pepper** to taste

Instructions

1. **Prepare the Salad Ingredients:** In a large salad bowl, combine the fresh arugula, sliced apple, chopped pecans, and optional ingredients like goat cheese and red onion.
2. **Make the Lemon Vinaigrette:** In a small bowl or jar, whisk together the olive oil, lemon juice, Dijon mustard, honey or maple syrup, and a pinch of salt and black pepper until well emulsified.
3. **Toss the Salad:** Drizzle the dressing over the salad mixture. Toss gently to coat the arugula and apples evenly with the dressing.
4. **Serve Immediately:** Divide the salad among four plates or bowls. Serve immediately to enjoy the fresh flavors and textures.

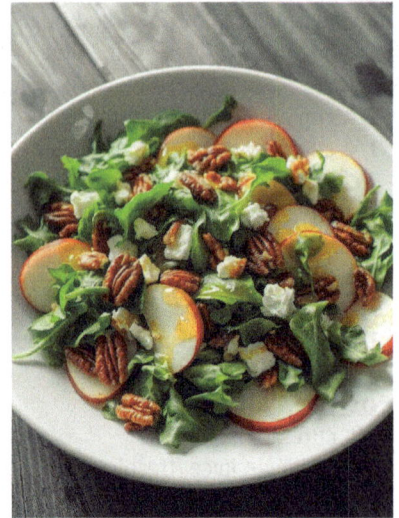

Nutritional Information (per serving)

- **Calories**: 210 kcal
- **Protein**: 4 g
- **Carbohydrates**: 18 g
- **Fats**: 16 g
- **Fiber**: 3 g
- **Cholesterol**: 10 mg (if cheese is used)
- **Sodium**: 150 mg
- **Potassium**: 280 mg

KALE & AVOCADO SALAD WITH LEMON-GINGER DRESSING

Yield: 4 servings • Preparation Time: 10 minutes • Cooking Time: None

Ingredients

> **4 cups** kale, stems removed and leaves chopped
> **1 ripe avocado**, diced
> **1 cup** cherry tomatoes, halved
> **1/2 cup** cucumber, diced
> **1/4 cup** red onion, thinly sliced
> **1/4 cup** pumpkin seeds (pepitas), toasted
> **1/4 cup** feta cheese, crumbled (optional)

For the Lemon-Ginger Dressing:

> **3 tbsp** extra virgin olive oil
> **2 tbsp** fresh lemon juice
> **1 tsp** fresh ginger, grated
> **1 tsp** honey or maple syrup (optional)
> **Salt and black pepper** to taste

Instructions

1. **Prepare the Kale:** In a large bowl, add the chopped kale. Massage the kale leaves with a little bit of olive oil and a pinch of salt for about 2 minutes until they start to soften and darken. This process makes the kale more tender and palatable.
2. **Add Salad Ingredients:** Add the diced avocado, halved cherry tomatoes, diced cucumber, sliced red onion, and toasted pumpkin seeds to the bowl with the kale. If using, add the crumbled feta cheese for a creamy touch.
3. **Make the Lemon-Ginger Dressing:** In a small bowl or jar, whisk together the olive oil, lemon juice, grated ginger, honey or maple syrup (if using), and a pinch of salt and black pepper until well combined.
4. **Dress the Salad:** Drizzle the dressing over the salad mixture. Toss gently to ensure the salad ingredients are evenly coated with the dressing.
5. **Serve Immediately:** Divide the salad among four plates or bowls. Enjoy this fresh and nutritious salad right away!

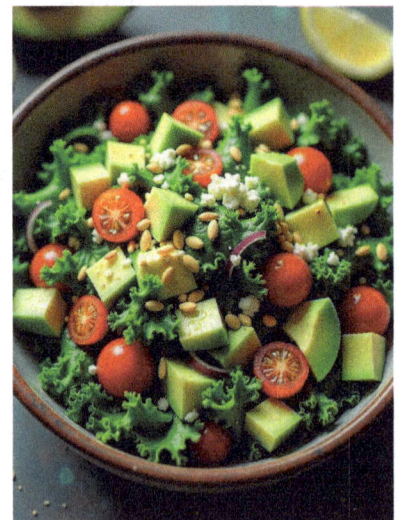

Nutritional Information (per serving)

- **Calories**: 280 kcal
- **Protein**: 6 g
- **Carbohydrates**: 20 g
- **Fats**: 22 g
- **Fiber**: 7 g
- **Cholesterol**: 5 mg (if cheese is used)
- **Sodium**: 180 mg
- **Potassium**: 450 mg

ROMAINE, CUCUMBER & DILL SALAD WITH OLIVE OIL

Yield: 4 servings • Preparation Time: 10 minutes • Cooking Time: None

Ingredients
> **4 cups** Romaine lettuce, chopped
> **1 medium cucumber**, sliced
> **1/4 cup** fresh dill, chopped
> **1/4 cup** red onion, thinly sliced
> **1/4 cup** cherry tomatoes, halved (optional)
> **1/4 cup** feta cheese, crumbled (optional)

For the Dressing:
> **3 tbsp** extra virgin olive oil
> **2 tbsp** apple cider vinegar
> **1 tsp** Dijon mustard
> **Salt and black pepper** to taste

Instructions
1. **Prepare the Vegetables:** In a large salad bowl, combine the chopped Romaine lettuce, sliced cucumber, chopped dill, and thinly sliced red onion. If using, add the halved cherry tomatoes and crumbled feta cheese for additional flavor and texture.
2. **Make the Dressing:** In a small bowl, whisk together the extra virgin olive oil, apple cider vinegar, Dijon mustard, and a pinch of salt and black pepper until well combined.
3. **Dress the Salad:** Drizzle the dressing over the salad ingredients. Toss gently to ensure all ingredients are coated with the dressing.
4. **Serve Immediately:** Divide the salad among four plates or bowls. Enjoy this refreshing salad right away!

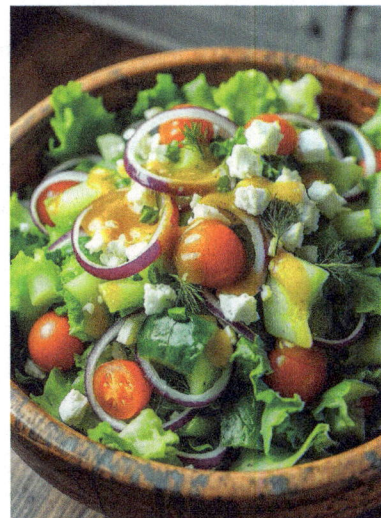

Nutritional Information (per serving)
- **Calories**: 150 kcal
- **Protein**: 4 g
- **Carbohydrates**: 8 g
- **Fats**: 12 g
- **Fiber**: 2 g
- **Cholesterol**: 10 mg (if cheese is used)
- **Sodium**: 200 mg
- **Potassium**: 300 mg

MIXED GREENS WITH GOLDEN BEETS AND POMEGRANATE SEEDS

Yield: 4 servings • Preparation Time: 15 minutes • Cooking Time: 30 minutes (plus cooling time)

Ingredients
> **4 cups** mixed greens (arugula, spinach, or baby kale)
> **2 medium golden beets**, peeled and diced
> **1 cup** pomegranate seeds (fresh or frozen)
> **1/4 cup** walnuts, chopped (optional)
> **1/4 cup** feta cheese, crumbled (optional)

For the Dressing:
> **3 tbsp** extra virgin olive oil
> **1 tbsp** balsamic vinegar
> **1 tsp** Dijon mustard
> **1 tsp** honey or maple syrup (optional)
> **Salt and black pepper** to taste

Instructions
1. **Preheat the Oven:** Preheat your oven to 400°F (200°C).
2. **Prepare the Golden Beets:** Wash and peel the golden beets. Cut them into small cubes (about 1/2 inch). Place the diced beets in a bowl and toss with 1 tbsp olive oil, salt, and black pepper.
3. **Roast the Beets:** Spread the beets in a single layer on a baking sheet lined with parchment paper. Roast in the preheated oven for 25-30 minutes, stirring halfway through. Remove from the oven and let cool.
4. **Prepare the Salad Base:** In a large bowl, add the mixed greens. Once the beets have cooled, add them on top of the greens along with the pomegranate seeds and walnuts (if using).
5. **Make the Dressing:** In a small bowl, whisk together the remaining olive oil, balsamic vinegar, Dijon mustard, honey (if using), and a pinch of salt and black pepper until well combined.
6. **Dress the Salad:** Drizzle the dressing over the salad and toss gently to combine all ingredients.

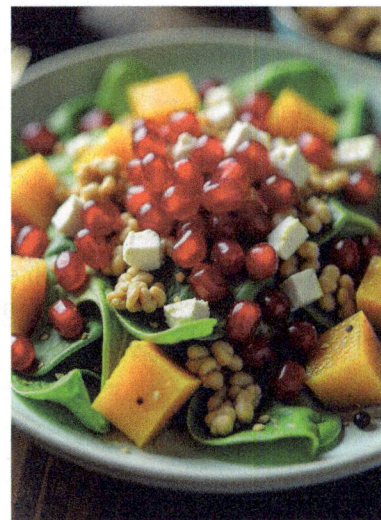

Nutritional Information (per serving)
- **Calories**: 180 kcal
- **Protein**: 4 g
- **Carbohydrates**: 12 g
- **Fats**: 15 g
- **Fiber**: 3 g
- **Cholesterol**: 10 mg (if cheese is used)
- **Sodium**: 150 mg
- **Potassium**: 400 mg

WATERCRESS & PEAR SALAD WITH HAZELNUTS

Yield: 4 servings • Preparation Time: 10 minutes • Cooking Time: 5 minutes (for toasting hazelnuts)

Ingredients
> **4 cups** watercress, washed and trimmed
> **2 ripe pears**, sliced (Bosc or Anjou pears work well)
> **1/2 cup** hazelnuts, chopped (raw or toasted)
> **1/4 cup** crumbled goat cheese (optional)

For the Dressing:
> **3 tbsp** extra virgin olive oil
> **1 tbsp** apple cider vinegar
> **1 tsp** Dijon mustard
> **1 tsp** honey (optional)
> **Salt and black pepper** to taste

Instructions
1. **Toast the Hazelnuts:** In a dry skillet over medium heat, toast the hazelnuts for about 3-5 minutes, stirring frequently, until fragrant and golden brown. Be careful not to burn them. Remove from heat and let cool.
2. **Prepare the Salad Base:** In a large bowl, add the watercress. Arrange the sliced pears on top and sprinkle with toasted hazelnuts.
3. **Make the Dressing:** In a small bowl, whisk together the olive oil, apple cider vinegar, Dijon mustard, honey (if using), salt, and black pepper until emulsified.
4. **Dress the Salad:** Drizzle the dressing over the salad and toss gently to combine all ingredients without bruising the pears.
5. **Serve Immediately:** Divide the salad among four plates or bowls. If desired, top with crumbled goat cheese for added flavor.

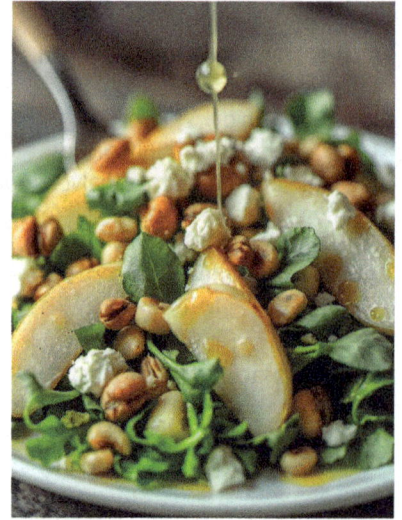

Nutritional Information (per serving)
- **Calories**: 180 kcal
- **Sodium**: 100 mg
- **Protein**: 4 g
- **Potassium**: 250 mg
- **Carbohydrates**: 16 g
- **Fats**: 12 g
- **Fiber**: 3 g
- **Cholesterol**: 5 mg (if cheese is used)

ENDIVE & WALNUT SALAD WITH POMEGRANATE DRESSING

Yield: 4 servings • Preparation Time: 15 minutes • Cooking Time: None

Ingredients
> **4 cups** endive, chopped (about 3 medium endives)
> **1 cup** walnuts, toasted and roughly chopped
> **1 cup** pomegranate seeds (from about 1 medium pomegranate)
> **1/4 cup** red onion, thinly sliced
> **1/4 cup** feta cheese, crumbled (optional)

For the Pomegranate Dressing:
> **1/4 cup** pomegranate juice (fresh or bottled)
> **2 tbsp** extra virgin olive oil
> **1 tbsp** apple cider vinegar
> **1 tsp** Dijon mustard
> **1 tsp** honey (optional)
> **Salt and black pepper** to taste

Instructions
1. **Prepare the Endive:** Wash the endive thoroughly and chop it into bite-sized pieces. Place the chopped endive in a large salad bowl.
2. **Toast the Walnuts:** In a dry skillet over medium heat, toast the walnuts for about 5 minutes, stirring frequently, until fragrant and lightly browned. Remove from heat and let cool slightly.
3. **Make the Dressing:** In a small bowl, whisk together the pomegranate juice, olive oil, apple cider vinegar, Dijon mustard, honey (if using), salt, and black pepper until well combined.
4. **Combine Ingredients:** Add the toasted walnuts, pomegranate seeds, and sliced red onion to the bowl with the endive. Toss gently to combine.
5. **Dress the Salad:** Drizzle the pomegranate dressing over the salad and toss gently to ensure everything is evenly coated.
6. **Serve Immediately**: Divide the salad among four plates or bowls. If desired, top each serving with crumbled feta cheese for added flavor.

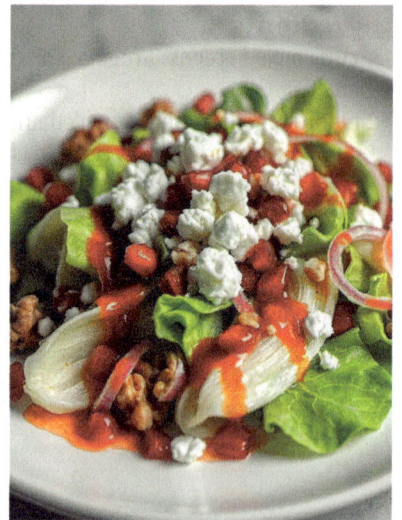

Nutritional Information (per serving)
- **Calories**: 230 kcal
- **Potassium**: 250 mg
- **Protein**: 6 g
- **Carbohydrates**: 14 g
- **Fats**: 18 g
- **Fiber**: 4 g
- **Cholesterol**: 10 mg
- **Sodium**: 120 mg

HEARTY & GRAIN SALADS

LENTIL & QUINOA SALAD WITH ROASTED RED PEPPERS

Yield: 4 servings • Preparation Time: 15 minutes • Cooking Time: 35 minutes

Ingredients
> **1/2 cup** dried green or brown lentils, rinsed
> **1/2 cup** quinoa, rinsed
> **1 1/2 cups** water or low-sodium vegetable broth, divided
> **1 medium** red bell pepper, roasted and diced
> **1/2 cup** cucumber, diced
> **1/4 cup** red onion, finely diced
> **1/4 cup** fresh parsley, chopped
> **1/4 cup** fresh cilantro, chopped
> **1/4 cup** crumbled feta cheese (optional, omit for vegan)

Dressing
> **3 tbsp** extra virgin olive oil
> **1 tbsp** apple cider vinegar
> **1 tbsp** lemon juice (freshly squeezed)
> **1 tsp** Dijon mustard
> **1/2 tsp** turmeric powder
> **Salt and black pepper** to taste

Optional Toppings
> **1/4 cup** toasted sunflower seeds or pumpkin seeds
> **2 tbsp** chopped fresh mint or basil

Instructions
1. **Cook the Lentils:** In a medium saucepan, add lentils and **1 cup** of water or vegetable broth. Bring to a boil, reduce heat, and let simmer for 20–25 minutes, or until lentils are tender but not mushy. Drain any excess liquid and let cool.
2. **Cook the Quinoa:** In a separate saucepan, combine quinoa and **1/2 cup** of water or vegetable broth. Bring to a boil, reduce heat, cover, and let simmer for 15–20 minutes, or until quinoa is fluffy and water is absorbed. Remove from heat and let cool slightly.
3. **Prepare the Dressing:** In a small bowl, whisk together olive oil, apple cider vinegar, lemon juice, Dijon mustard, turmeric powder, and a pinch of salt and black pepper until smooth and well-combined.
4. **Assemble the Salad:** In a large bowl, combine cooked lentils, quinoa, roasted red pepper, cucumber, red onion, parsley, and cilantro. Pour the dressing over the salad and toss gently to coat.
5. **Serve and Garnish:** Divide the salad among four bowls. Top with crumbled feta cheese if using, and sprinkle with toasted sunflower seeds or pumpkin seeds for added texture. Garnish with fresh mint or basil if desired.

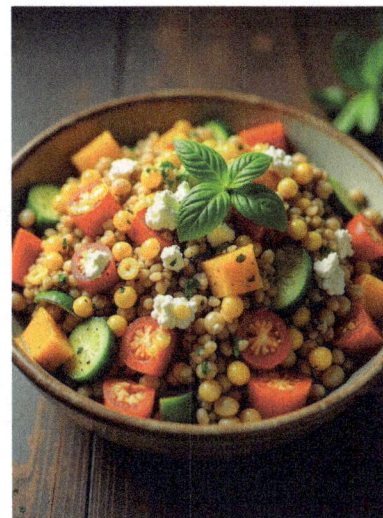

Nutritional Information (per serving)
- **Calories**: 320 kcal
- **Protein**: 10 g
- **Carbohydrates**: 35 g
- **Fats**: 15 g
- **Fiber**: 8 g
- **Cholesterol**: 0 mg
- **Sodium**: 120 mg
- **Potassium**: 500 mg

WILD RICE & BLUEBERRY SALAD WITH SPINACH

Yield: 4 servings • Preparation Time: 15 minutes • Cooking Time: 40 minutes (includes wild rice cooking time)

Ingredients
Salad
> **1 cup** wild rice, uncooked
> **3 cups** fresh baby spinach, roughly chopped
> **1 cup** fresh blueberries
> **1/2 cup** cucumber, diced
> **1/4 cup** red onion, finely chopped
> **1/4 cup** almonds, sliced or slivered (optional for crunch and extra healthy fats)

Dressing
> **3 tbsp** extra-virgin olive oil
> **2 tbsp** apple cider vinegar
> **1 tbsp** fresh lemon juice
> **1 tsp** maple syrup or honey
> **1/2 tsp** Dijon mustard
> **Salt and black pepper**, to taste

Optional Add-Ins
> **1 tbsp** chia seeds or hemp seeds for additional omega-3s
> **1/4 cup** crumbled feta for added creaminess and flavor (optional)

Instructions
1. **Cook the Wild Rice:** In a medium saucepan, combine wild rice with 2 1/2 cups of water and a pinch of salt. Bring to a boil, then reduce the heat to low, cover, and simmer for 35–40 minutes, or until the rice is tender and the water is absorbed. Drain any excess water, fluff with a fork, and set aside to cool.
2. **Prepare the Dressing:** In a small bowl, whisk together olive oil, apple cider vinegar, lemon juice, maple syrup, and Dijon mustard. Season with salt and pepper to taste and set aside.
3. **Assemble the Salad:** In a large mixing bowl, combine the cooked wild rice, spinach, blueberries, cucumber, red onion, and almonds (if using). Pour the dressing over the salad and toss gently until all ingredients are well coated.
4. **Serve and Garnish:** Divide the salad into four servings. Top with optional add-ins like chia seeds or crumbled feta, if desired.

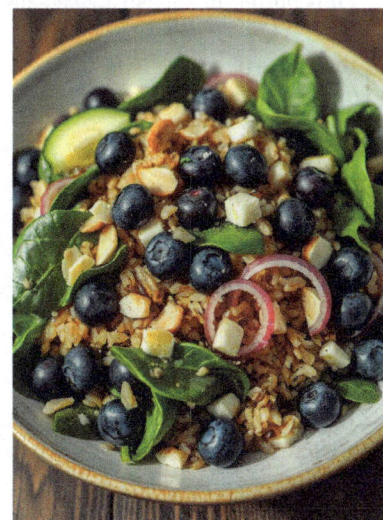

Nutritional Information (per serving)
- **Calories**: 300 kcal
- **Protein**: 6 g
- **Carbohydrates**: 40 g
- **Fats**: 13 g
- **Fiber**: 6 g
- **Cholesterol**: 0 mg
- **Sodium**: 80 mg
- **Potassium**: 410 mg

MILLET & ZUCCHINI SALAD WITH FRESH BASIL

Yield: 4 servings • Preparation Time: 15 minutes • Cooking Time: 20 minutes (includes millet cooking time)

Ingredients
Salad
> **1 cup** millet, uncooked
> **2 medium zucchinis**, diced or spiralized
> **1/2 cup** cherry tomatoes, halved
> **1/4 cup** fresh basil leaves, chopped
> **1/4 cup** cucumber, diced
> **1/4 cup** red bell pepper, finely diced
> **2 tbsp** red onion, finely chopped (optional for flavor)

Dressing
> **3 tbsp** extra-virgin olive oil
> **1 tbsp** fresh lemon juice
> **1 tsp** apple cider vinegar
> **1/2 tsp** honey or maple syrup
> **1 clove** garlic, minced
> **Salt and black pepper**, to taste

Optional Add-Ins
> **2 tbsp** pumpkin seeds or sunflower seeds for crunch
> **1/4 cup** crumbled feta or goat cheese for added creaminess (optional)

Instructions
1. **Cook the Millet:** In a medium saucepan, combine millet with 2 cups of water and a pinch of salt. Bring to a boil over medium-high heat, then reduce the heat to low, cover, and simmer for 15–20 minutes, or until the millet is tender and the water is absorbed. Remove from heat and set aside to cool.
2. **Prepare the Dressing:** In a small bowl, whisk together olive oil, lemon juice, apple cider vinegar, honey, and minced garlic. Season with salt and pepper to taste and set aside.
3. **Assemble the Salad:** In a large mixing bowl, combine the cooled millet, zucchini, cherry tomatoes, basil, cucumber, red bell pepper, and red onion (if using). Pour the dressing over the salad and toss gently to coat all the ingredients.
4. **Serve and Garnish:** Divide the salad into four servings. Top with optional add-ins like pumpkin seeds or crumbled feta for extra flavor and texture, if desired.

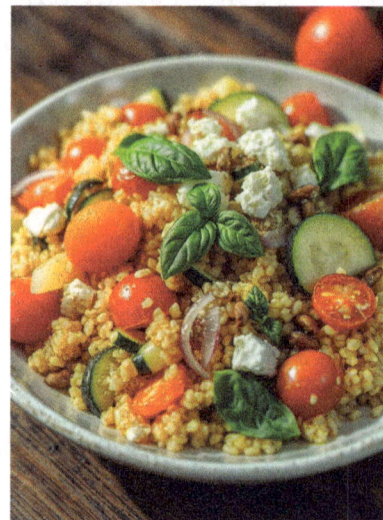

Nutritional Information (per serving)
- **Calories**: 280 kcal
- **Protein**: 6 g
- **Carbohydrates**: 38 g
- **Fats**: 12 g
- **Fiber**: 5 g
- **Cholesterol**: 0 mg
- **Sodium**: 60 mg
- **Potassium**: 420 mg

QUINOA & ROASTED BUTTERNUT SQUASH SALAD

Yield: 4 servings • Preparation Time: 15 minutes • Cooking Time: 30 minutes

Ingredients
Salad
> **1 cup** quinoa, uncooked
> **2 cups** butternut squash, peeled and cubed (1/2-inch pieces)
> **1 tbsp** olive oil
> **1/4 tsp** sea salt
> **1/4 tsp** black pepper
> **2 cups** mixed greens (such as spinach and arugula)
> **1/4 cup** pomegranate seeds
> **1/4 cup** walnuts, toasted and chopped
> **2 tbsp** fresh parsley, chopped (optional)

Lemon-Tahini Dressing
> **2 tbsp** tahini
> **2 tbsp** fresh lemon juice
> **1 tbsp** apple cider vinegar
> **1 tbsp** maple syrup or honey
> **2 tbsp** water (or more for desired consistency)
> **1/4 tsp** sea salt
> **1 clove** garlic, minced

Instructions
1. **Prepare the Quinoa:** Rinse quinoa under cold water. In a medium saucepan, combine quinoa with 2 cups of water. Bring to a boil over medium-high heat, then reduce the heat to low, cover, and simmer for 15 minutes, or until the quinoa is tender and water is absorbed. Fluff with a fork and set aside to cool.
2. **Roast the Butternut Squash:** Preheat your oven to 400°F (200°C). Place butternut squash cubes on a baking sheet, drizzle with olive oil, and season with salt and pepper. Toss to coat, then spread in a single layer. Roast for 25–30 minutes, flipping halfway through, until the squash is tender and caramelized. Remove from oven and let cool.
3. **Prepare the Dressing:** In a small bowl, whisk together tahini, lemon juice, apple cider vinegar, maple syrup, water, sea salt, and minced garlic until smooth. Adjust water as needed for desired consistency.
4. **Assemble the Salad:** In a large mixing bowl, combine the cooked quinoa, roasted butternut squash, mixed greens, pomegranate seeds, and toasted walnuts. Drizzle with the dressing and toss gently to combine. Top with fresh parsley if desired.
5. **Serve:** Divide into four servings. Enjoy warm or at room temperature.

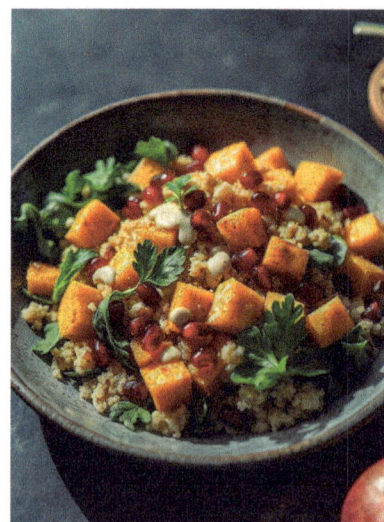

Nutritional Information (per serving)
- **Calories**: 340 kcal
- **Protein**: 8 g
- **Carbohydrates**: 45 g
- **Fats**: 14 g
- **Fiber**: 6 g
- **Cholesterol**: 0 mg
- **Sodium**: 120 mg
- **Potassium**: 550 mg

SWEET POTATO & BLACK BEAN ANTI-INFLAMMATORY SALAD

Yield: 4 servings • Preparation Time: 15 minutes • Cooking Time: 30 minutes

Ingredients
Salad
> **2 medium** sweet potatoes (about 1 lb), peeled and diced into 1/2-inch cubes
> **1 can (15 oz)** black beans, rinsed and drained
> **1 red bell pepper**, diced
> **1 cup** corn (fresh, frozen, or canned)
> **1/2 cup** red onion, finely chopped
> **2 cups** fresh spinach or kale, chopped
> **1 avocado**, diced
> **1 tbsp** olive oil
> **1/2 tsp** sea salt
> **1/2 tsp** black pepper
> **1/2 tsp** smoked paprika (optional)
> **1/4 tsp** cayenne pepper (optional)

Cilantro-Lime Dressing
> **3 tbsp** olive oil
> **2 tbsp** fresh lime juice
> **1 tbsp** apple cider vinegar
> **1 tsp** honey or maple syrup
> **1/4 cup** fresh cilantro, chopped
> **1/2 tsp** ground cumin
> **1/4 tsp** sea salt
> **1/4 tsp** black pepper

Instructions
1. **Roast the Sweet Potatoes:** Preheat your oven to 400°F (200°C). On a baking sheet, toss the diced sweet potatoes with 1 tbsp olive oil, sea salt, black pepper, and optional smoked paprika and cayenne pepper. Spread them in a single layer. Roast in the preheated oven for 25–30 minutes, or until tender and slightly caramelized, stirring halfway through. Remove from oven and let cool.
2. **Prepare the Dressing:** In a small bowl, whisk together the olive oil, lime juice, apple cider vinegar, honey (or maple syrup), chopped cilantro, cumin, sea salt, and black pepper until well combined.
3. **Assemble the Salad:** In a large mixing bowl, combine the roasted sweet potatoes, black beans, diced red bell pepper, corn, red onion, and chopped greens (spinach or kale). Drizzle the cilantro-lime dressing over the salad and toss gently to combine.
4. **Add Avocado:** Just before serving, gently fold in the diced avocado to maintain its shape.
5. **Serve:** Divide the salad into four serving bowls and enjoy immediately, or refrigerate for up to 1 day before serving.

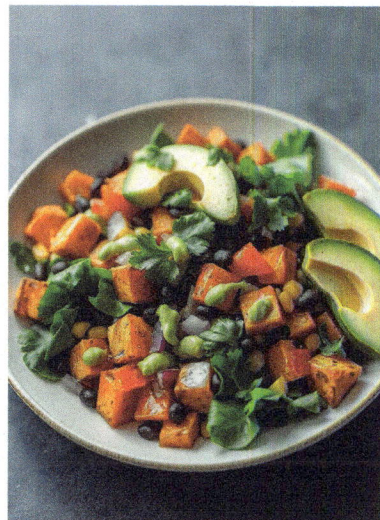

Nutritional Information (per serving)
- **Calories**: 330 kcal
- **Protein**: 10 g
- **Carbohydrates**: 45 g
- **Fats**: 14 g
- **Fiber**: 10 g
- **Cholesterol**: 0 mg
- **Sodium**: 260 mg
- **Potassium**: 750 mg

BULGUR SALAD WITH CUCUMBER, PARSLEY & MINT

Yield: 4 servings • Preparation Time: 15 minutes • Cooking Time: 15 minutes (includes passive soaking time)

Ingredients
Salad
> **1 cup** bulgur wheat
> **2 cups** water or vegetable broth
> **1 medium** cucumber, diced
> **1 cup** cherry tomatoes, halved
> **1/2 cup** red onion, finely chopped
> **1 cup** fresh parsley, chopped
> **1/2 cup** fresh mint, chopped
> **1/4 cup** olive oil
> **1/4 tsp** sea salt (or to taste)
> **1/4 tsp** black pepper (or to taste)
> **1/2 tsp** ground cumin (optional)

Dressing
> **2 tbsp** fresh lemon juice
> **1 tbsp** apple cider vinegar
> **1/2 tsp** honey or maple syrup (optional)
> **1/4 tsp** sea salt
> **1/4 tsp** black pepper

Instructions
1. **Prepare the Bulgur:** In a medium saucepan, bring 2 cups of water or vegetable broth to a boil. Stir in the 1 cup of bulgur wheat, cover, and remove from heat. Let it sit for about 15 minutes, or until the bulgur is tender and the liquid is absorbed. Fluff with a fork once done.
2. **Prepare the Vegetables and Herbs:** While the bulgur is soaking, chop the cucumber, cherry tomatoes, red onion, parsley, and mint.
3. **Make the Dressing:** In a small bowl, whisk together the 2 tbsp lemon juice, 1 tbsp apple cider vinegar, 1/2 tsp honey (or maple syrup), 1/4 tsp sea salt, and 1/4 tsp black pepper.
4. **Combine Ingredients:** In a large mixing bowl, combine the cooked bulgur, diced cucumber, halved cherry tomatoes, chopped red onion, parsley, and mint. Drizzle the 1/4 cup olive oil and the prepared dressing over the salad, then sprinkle with 1/2 tsp ground cumin, 1/4 tsp sea salt, and 1/4 tsp black pepper. Toss gently to combine.
5. **Serve:** Taste and adjust seasoning as needed. Serve immediately or let it chill in the refrigerator for about 30 minutes to enhance the flavors.

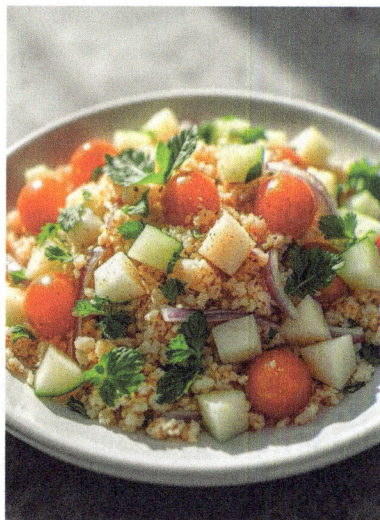

Nutritional Information (per serving)
- **Calories**: 230
- **Protein**: 6g
- **Carbohydrates**: 34g
- **Fats**: 10g
- **Fiber**: 6g
- **Cholesterol**: 0mg
- **Sodium**: 150mg (adjust based on added salt)
- **Potassium**: 450mg

4. GRAINS, PASTA, AND RICE RECIPES
WHOLE GRAINS

BARLEY & MUSHROOM RISOTTO

Yield: 4 servings • Preparation Time: 15 minutes • Cooking Time: 35 minutes

Ingredients
Risotto
› **1 cup** pearl barley, rinsed
› **4 cups** vegetable broth (low-sodium)
› **1 medium** onion, finely chopped
› **2 cloves** garlic, minced
› **8 oz** mushrooms (such as cremini or shiitake), sliced
› **1 tbsp** olive oil
› **1 tbsp** fresh thyme leaves (or **1 tsp** dried thyme)
› **1/2 cup** nutritional yeast (for a cheesy flavor, optional)
› **Salt and black pepper to taste**
› **1 cup** fresh spinach, chopped (optional)

Toppings
› **1/4 cup** fresh parsley, chopped
› **2 tbsp** toasted pine nuts or walnuts (for crunch)

Instructions
1. **Prepare the Broth:** In a medium saucepan, bring 4 cups of vegetable broth to a gentle simmer over low heat. Keep it warm while you prepare the risotto.
2. **Sauté the Aromatics:** In a large skillet or pot, heat 1 tbsp of olive oil over medium heat. Add the finely chopped 1 medium onion and sauté for about 5 minutes until it becomes translucent. Stir in 2 cloves minced garlic and continue to sauté for another 1-2 minutes until fragrant.
3. **Cook the Mushrooms:** Add 8 oz sliced mushrooms to the skillet and cook for about 5-7 minutes until they are tender and their moisture has evaporated.
4. **Toast the Barley:** Stir in the rinsed 1 cup pearl barley, ensuring it is well coated with the oil and mushroom mixture.
5. **Add Broth Gradually:** Gradually add the warm vegetable broth, one ladle at a time, stirring frequently. Allow the barley to absorb the broth before adding more. Continue this process for about 30 minutes, or until the barley is tender but still has a slight bite.
6. **Season the Risotto:** Once the barley is cooked, incorporate 1 tbsp fresh thyme leaves (or 1 tsp dried thyme) and 1/2 cup nutritional yeast for added flavor. Season with salt and black pepper to taste. If using, fold in 1 cup fresh spinach until it wilts.
7. **Serve:** Divide the risotto among four bowls. Top each bowl with 1/4 cup fresh parsley and 2 tbsp toasted pine nuts or walnuts for a delightful crunch.

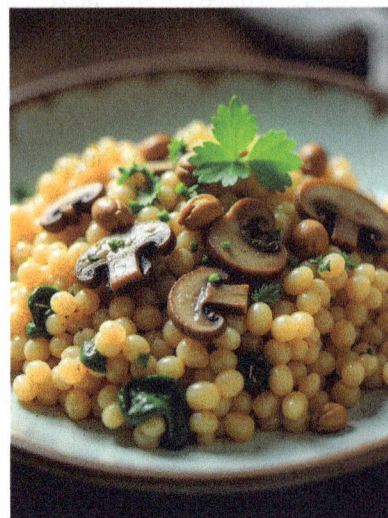

Nutritional Information (per serving)
- **Calories**: 290 kcal
- **Protein**: 9 g
- **Carbohydrates**: 49 g
- **Fats**: 7 g
- **Fiber**: 8 g
- **Cholesterol**: 0 mg
- **Sodium**: 150 mg (adjust based on broth used)
- **Potassium**: 550 mg

LEMON & HERB QUINOA WITH ROASTED VEGETABLES

Yield: 4 servings • Preparation Time: 15 minutes • Cooking Time: 30 minutes

Ingredients
Quinoa
› **1 cup** quinoa, rinsed
› **2 cups** vegetable broth (low-sodium)
› **1 tbsp** olive oil
› **1/4 tsp** sea salt
› **1/4 tsp** black pepper
› **1/2 tsp** garlic powder

Roasted Vegetables
› **1 medium** zucchini, diced
› **1 red bell pepper, diced**
› **1 cup** cherry tomatoes, halved
› **1 small red onion, diced**
› **1 tbsp** olive oil
› **1/2 tsp** dried oregano
› **1/2 tsp** dried thyme
› **Salt and black pepper to taste**

Lemon Herb Dressing
› **2 tbsp** fresh lemon juice
› **1 tbsp** olive oil
› **1 tsp** Dijon mustard
› **1 clove** garlic, minced
› **1/4 cup** fresh parsley, chopped
› **1/4 cup** fresh basil, chopped (optional)
› Salt and black pepper to taste

Instructions
1. **Roast the Vegetables:** Preheat your oven to 425°F (220°C). In a large bowl, combine 1 medium zucchini, diced, 1 red bell pepper, diced, 1 cup cherry tomatoes, halved, and 1 small red onion, diced. Drizzle with 1 tbsp olive oil, and sprinkle with 1/2 tsp dried oregano, 1/2 tsp dried thyme, and salt and black pepper to taste. Toss until the vegetables are evenly coated. Spread them on a baking sheet in a single layer. Roast in the preheated oven for about 20-25 minutes, or until the vegetables are tender and slightly caramelized, stirring halfway through.
2. **Cook the Quinoa:** While the vegetables are roasting, combine 1 cup quinoa with 2 cups vegetable broth, 1 tbsp olive oil, 1/4 tsp sea salt, 1/4 tsp black pepper, and 1/2 tsp garlic powder in a medium saucepan. Bring to a boil over medium-high heat, then reduce the heat to low. Cover and simmer for about 15 minutes, or until the quinoa is fluffy and the liquid is absorbed. Remove from heat and let it sit covered for an additional 5 minutes, then fluff with a fork.
3. **Prepare the Dressing:** In a small bowl, whisk together 2 tbsp fresh lemon juice, 1 tbsp olive oil, 1 tsp Dijon mustard, 1 clove minced garlic, 1/4 cup chopped fresh parsley, and 1/4 cup chopped fresh basil (if using). Season with salt and black pepper to taste.
4. **Combine the Quinoa and Vegetables:** In a large mixing bowl, combine the cooked quinoa and roasted vegetables. Drizzle with the lemon herb dressing and toss gently to combine.
5. **Serve:** Divide the quinoa and vegetable mixture among four serving plates. Enjoy warm or at room temperature.

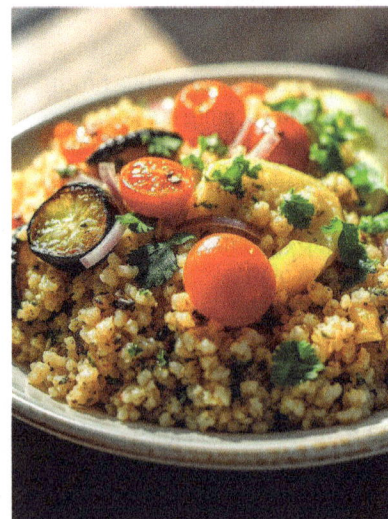

Nutritional Information (per serving)
- **Calories**: 290 kcal
- **Protein**: 9 g
- **Carbohydrates**: 41 g
- **Fats**: 12 g
- **Fiber**: 7 g
- **Cholesterol**: 0 mg
- **Sodium**: 200 mg (adjust based on broth used)
- **Potassium**: 550 mg

COCONUT & GINGER MILLET WITH CARROTS

Yield: 4 servings • Preparation Time: 10 minutes • Cooking Time: 25 minutes

Ingredients
Millet
> **1 cup** millet, rinsed
> **2 cups** coconut milk (light or regular)
> **1 cup** water
> **1/2 tsp** sea salt

Vegetables
> **2 cups** carrots, peeled and sliced (or diced)
> **1 tbsp** fresh ginger, grated
> **1 tbsp** olive oil
> **1/2 tsp** turmeric powder
> **1/4 tsp** black pepper
> **1/4 tsp** cayenne pepper (optional, for heat)

Garnish
> **1/4 cup** fresh cilantro, chopped (optional)
> **1/4 cup** toasted coconut flakes (optional)
> **Juice of 1 lime** (optional)

Instructions
1. **Prepare the Millet:** In a medium saucepan, combine 1 cup rinsed millet, 2 cups coconut milk, 1 cup water, and 1/2 tsp sea salt. Bring to a boil over medium-high heat, then reduce the heat to low. Cover and simmer for about 20 minutes, or until the millet is tender and the liquid is absorbed. Remove from heat and let it sit, covered, for an additional 5 minutes. Fluff the millet with a fork and set aside.
2. **Cook the Carrots:** In a large skillet, heat 1 tbsp olive oil over medium heat. Add the 2 cups sliced carrots and sauté for about 5 minutes, or until they start to soften. Stir in the 1 tbsp grated ginger, 1/2 tsp turmeric powder, 1/4 tsp black pepper, and 1/4 tsp cayenne pepper (if using). Continue to cook for another 3–4 minutes, or until the carrots are tender.
3. **Combine and Serve:** Add the cooked millet to the skillet with the carrots and spices. Stir to combine and heat through for a couple of minutes. Adjust seasoning as needed. If desired, add the juice of 1 lime for a fresh flavor boost.
4. **Garnish:** Divide the Coconut & Ginger Millet with Carrots among serving bowls. Top with chopped fresh cilantro and toasted coconut flakes for extra flavor and texture.

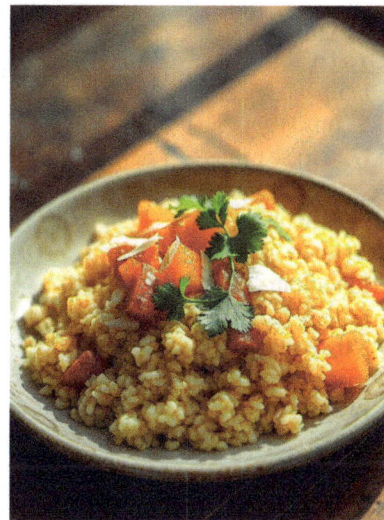

Nutritional Information (per serving)
- **Calories**: 320 kcal
- **Fiber**: 6 g
- **Protein**: 7 g
- **Cholesterol**: 0 mg
- **Carbohydrates**: 50 g
- **Sodium**: 280 mg
- **Fats**: 12 g
- **Potassium**: 450 mg

GOLDEN FARRO WITH SWEET POTATOES & SAGE

Yield: 4 servings • Preparation Time: 15 minutes • Cooking Time: 35 minutes

Ingredients
Grain
> **1 cup** farro, rinsed
> **3 cups** vegetable broth or water
> **1/2 tsp** sea salt

Vegetables
> **2 cups** sweet potatoes, peeled and diced (about 1/2-inch cubes)
> **2 tbsp** olive oil
> **1/2 tsp** black pepper
> **1/2 tsp** garlic powder (optional)
> **1/2 tsp** smoked paprika (optional)

Herbs
> **2 tbsp** fresh sage, chopped (or 1 tbsp dried sage)
> **1/2 cup** onion, finely chopped
> **1/4 cup** walnuts, chopped (optional for crunch)

Instructions
1. **Cook the Farro:** In a medium saucepan, combine 1 cup farro, 3 cups vegetable broth (or water), and 1/2 tsp sea salt. Bring to a boil over medium-high heat, then reduce the heat to low. Cover and simmer for about 25–30 minutes, or until the farro is tender and the liquid is absorbed. Remove from heat and let it sit, covered, for an additional 5 minutes. Fluff with a fork and set aside.
2. **Roast the Sweet Potatoes:** Preheat your oven to 425°F (220°C). On a baking sheet, toss the 2 cups diced sweet potatoes with 2 tbsp olive oil, 1/2 tsp black pepper, 1/2 tsp garlic powder, and 1/2 tsp smoked paprika (if using). Spread the sweet potatoes in a single layer and roast for about 25 minutes, or until they are tender and slightly caramelized, flipping halfway through. Remove from the oven and let cool slightly.
3. **Sauté the Onions and Sage:** In a large skillet, heat a little olive oil over medium heat. Add the 1/2 cup chopped onion and cook for about 5 minutes, or until translucent. Stir in the 2 tbsp chopped fresh sage and cook for another 1–2 minutes until fragrant.
4. **Combine Ingredients:** Add the roasted sweet potatoes and cooked farro to the skillet with the onions and sage. Stir to combine and heat through for a couple of minutes. Adjust seasoning as needed.
5. **Serve:** Divide the Golden Farro with Sweet Potatoes & Sage among serving bowls. If desired, top with chopped walnuts for added crunch and nutrition.

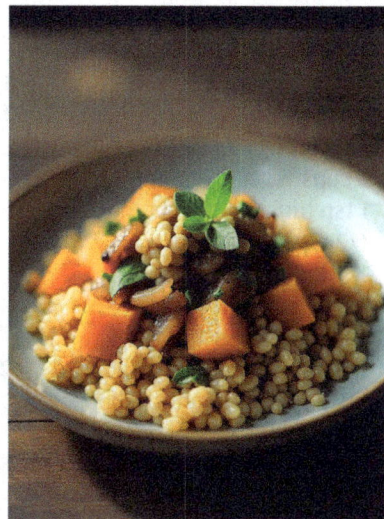

Nutritional Information (per serving)
- **Calories**: 320 kcal
- **Fiber**: 8 g
- **Protein**: 8 g
- **Cholesterol**: 0 mg
- **Carbohydrates**: 50 g
- **Sodium**: 300 mg
- **Fats**: 12 g
- **Potassium**: 550 mg

WILD RICE PILAF WITH CRANBERRIES AND PECANS

Yield: 4 servings • Preparation Time: 10 minutes • Cooking Time:40 minutes

Ingredients
Grain
› **1 cup** wild rice, rinsed
› **3 cups** vegetable broth or water
› **1/2 tsp** sea salt

Vegetables
› **1 small** onion, finely chopped
› **2 cloves** garlic, minced
› **1 medium** carrot, diced
› **1** celery stalk, diced
› **2 tbsp** olive oil

Fruits & Nuts
› **1/2 cup** dried cranberries (unsweetened if possible)
› **1/2 cup** pecans, roughly chopped (can be toasted for added flavor)

Herbs & Seasonings
› **1/2 tsp** dried thyme
› **1/2 tsp** dried rosemary
› **1/4 tsp** black pepper
› **1/4 tsp** red pepper flakes (optional for a bit of heat)
› **2 tbsp** fresh parsley, chopped (for garnish)

Instructions
1. **Cook the Wild Rice:** In a medium saucepan, combine 1 cup wild rice, 3 cups vegetable broth, and 1/2 tsp sea salt. Bring to a boil over medium-high heat, then reduce the heat to low, cover, and simmer for about 35–40 minutes, or until the rice is tender and the grains have split. Remove from heat and let sit covered for an additional 5 minutes, then fluff with a fork.
2. **Sauté the Vegetables:** While the rice is cooking, heat 2 tbsp olive oil in a large skillet over medium heat. Add the 1 small chopped onion and sauté for about 5 minutes until translucent. Stir in the 2 minced garlic cloves, 1 diced carrot, and 1 diced celery stalk. Cook for another 5-7 minutes, stirring occasionally, until the vegetables are softened.
3. **Combine Ingredients:** Once the wild rice is cooked, add it to the skillet with the sautéed vegetables. Stir in the 1/2 cup dried cranberries, 1/2 cup chopped pecans, 1/2 tsp dried thyme, 1/2 tsp dried rosemary, 1/4 tsp black pepper, and 1/4 tsp red pepper flakes (if using). Mix well to combine all ingredients and heat through for another 2–3 minutes.
4. **Serve:** Remove from heat and transfer the pilaf to a serving dish. Garnish with 2 tbsp fresh parsley before serving.

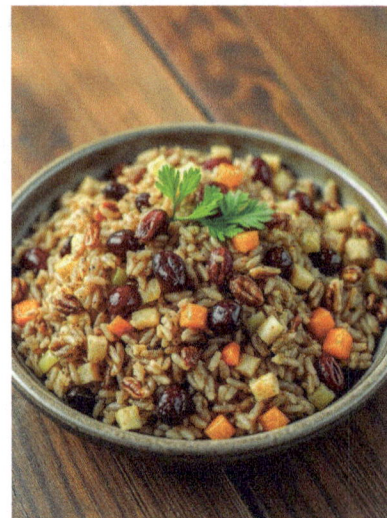

Nutritional Information (per serving)
- **Calories**: 290 kcal
- **Protein**: 8 g
- **Carbohydrates**: 40 g
- **Fats**: 12 g
- **Fiber**: 6 g
- **Cholesterol**: 0 mg
- **Sodium**: 350 mg
- **Potassium**: 450 mg

TURMERIC-SPICED BULGUR WITH MIXED HERBS

Yield: 4 servings • Preparation Time: 10 minutes • Cooking Time: 15 minutes

Ingredients
Bulgur
› **1 cup** bulgur wheat, rinsed
› **2 cups** vegetable broth or water
› **1 tsp** turmeric powder
› **1/2 tsp** ground cumin
› **1/4 tsp** sea salt
› **1 tbsp** olive oil

Mixed Herbs
› **1/4 cup** fresh parsley, chopped
› **1/4 cup** fresh cilantro, chopped
› **1/4 cup** fresh dill or mint, chopped
› **1 clove** garlic, minced (optional)

Optional Add-Ins
› **1/2 cup** diced bell peppers (any color)
› **1/2 cup** chopped spinach or kale
› **1/4 cup** toasted pine nuts or slivered almonds

Instructions
1. **Cook the Bulgur:** In a medium saucepan, combine 1 cup rinsed bulgur, 2 cups vegetable broth, 1 tsp turmeric powder, 1/2 tsp ground cumin, and 1/4 tsp sea salt. Bring the mixture to a boil over medium-high heat. Once boiling, reduce the heat to low, cover, and simmer for about 12-15 minutes until the bulgur is tender and has absorbed the liquid. Remove from heat and let it sit, covered, for another 5 minutes.
2. **Fluff the Bulgur:** After the bulgur has rested, use a fork to fluff it, breaking up any clumps. Drizzle 1 tbsp olive oil over the bulgur and stir to combine.
3. **Prepare the Mixed Herbs**: In a large mixing bowl, combine the 1/4 cup chopped parsley, 1/4 cup chopped cilantro, 1/4 cup chopped dill or mint, and 1 clove minced garlic (if using). If you are adding diced bell peppers or chopped spinach, include them in this step as well.
4. **Combine and Serve:** Add the fluffed bulgur to the bowl of herbs and vegetables. Toss gently to mix all the ingredients well, allowing the flavors to combine. Adjust seasoning with additional salt and pepper to taste.
5. **Serve:** Transfer the turmeric-spiced bulgur to a serving dish. Optionally, top with toasted pine nuts or slivered almonds for added crunch and nutrition. Enjoy warm or at room temperature.

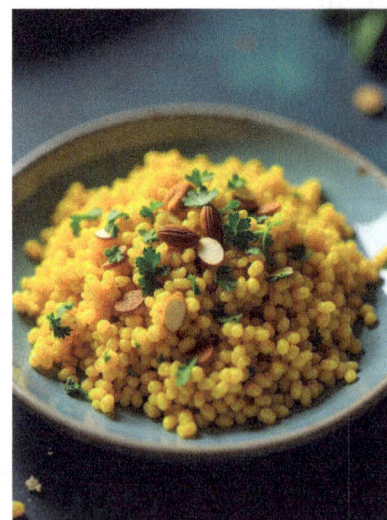

Nutritional Information (per serving)
- **Calories**: 210 kcal
- **Protein**: 7 g
- **Carbohydrates**: 35 g
- **Fats**: 7 g
- **Fiber**: 6 g
- **Cholesterol**: 0 mg
- **Sodium**: 220 mg
- **Potassium**: 350 mg

PASTA & NOODLES

CHICKPEA PASTA WITH SPINACH & WALNUT PESTO

Yield: 4 servings • Preparation Time: 15 minutes • Cooking Time: 10 minutes

Ingredients
Pasta
› **8 oz** chickpea pasta (such as penne or fusilli)
› **1/4 tsp** sea salt

Walnut Pesto
› **1 1/2 cups** fresh spinach, packed
› **1/2 cup** fresh basil leaves
› **1/2 cup** walnuts, toasted
› **1 clove** garlic, minced
› **1/4 cup** extra-virgin olive oil
› **2 tbsp** nutritional yeast or grated Parmesan (optional)
› **1 tbsp** fresh lemon juice
› **1/4 tsp** sea salt
› **1/4 tsp** black pepper

Optional Add-Ins
› **1/2 cup** cherry tomatoes, halved
› **1/4 cup** sun-dried tomatoes, chopped
› **1/4 cup** pine nuts, toasted (for added crunch)

Instructions
1. **Cook the Pasta:** In a large pot of boiling salted water, cook the chickpea pasta according to package instructions until al dente, about 8-10 minutes. Drain and set aside.
2. **Prepare the Walnut Pesto:** In a food processor, combine 1 1/2 cups fresh spinach, 1/2 cup fresh basil leaves, 1/2 cup toasted walnuts, 1 minced garlic clove, 1/4 cup extra-virgin olive oil, 2 tbsp nutritional yeast or Parmesan (if using), 1 tbsp lemon juice, 1/4 tsp sea salt, and 1/4 tsp black pepper. Process until smooth and creamy, scraping down the sides as needed. Adjust seasoning to taste.
3. **Combine the Pasta and Pesto:** In a large mixing bowl, combine the cooked chickpea pasta and the spinach walnut pesto. Toss well to coat the pasta evenly. Add cherry tomatoes or sun-dried tomatoes if desired.
4. **Serve:** Divide into four servings and top with additional toasted pine nuts or a sprinkle of nutritional yeast for extra flavor and texture.

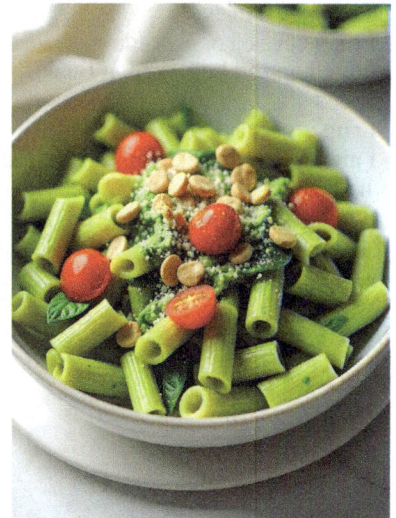

Nutritional Information (per serving)
- **Calories**: 420 kcal
- **Protein**: 15 g
- **Carbohydrates**: 32 g
- **Fats**: 24 g
- **Fiber**: 8 g
- **Cholesterol**: 0 mg
- **Sodium**: 180 mg
- **Potassium**: 520 mg

ZUCCHINI NOODLES WITH BASIL, TOMATO & GARLIC

Yield: 4 servings • Preparation Time: 15 minutes • Cooking Time: 5 minutes

Ingredients
Noodles
› **4 medium zucchini**, spiralized (about 6 cups of noodles)
› **1/4 tsp** sea salt

Sauce
› **1 tbsp** extra-virgin olive oil
› **3 cloves garlic**, minced
› **1 1/2 cups** cherry tomatoes, halved
› **1/2 cup** fresh basil leaves, chopped
› **1 tbsp** fresh lemon juice
› **1/4 tsp** black pepper

Optional Add-Ins
› **1/4 cup** sun-dried tomatoes, chopped
› **2 tbsp** nutritional yeast or grated Parmesan (optional)
› **1/4 tsp** red pepper flakes for a touch of heat

Instructions
1. **Prepare the Zucchini Noodles:** Spiralize the zucchini into noodles using a spiralizer or julienne peeler. Place the zucchini noodles in a colander and sprinkle with 1/4 tsp sea salt to help release excess water. Let sit for 5 minutes.
2. **Sauté the Garlic and Tomatoes:** In a large skillet, heat 1 tbsp olive oil over medium heat. Add 3 minced garlic cloves and sauté for 1-2 minutes until fragrant but not browned. Add 1 1/2 cups cherry tomatoes and cook for 2-3 minutes, stirring occasionally until tomatoes soften slightly.
3. **Add Zucchini Noodles and Basil:** Gently pat the zucchini noodles dry with a paper towel to remove any moisture. Add the noodles to the skillet, along with 1/2 cup chopped basil. Toss well to combine with the garlic and tomatoes, cooking for 1-2 minutes until warmed through but still slightly crisp.
4. **Finish with Lemon and Seasoning:** Drizzle the noodles with 1 tbsp fresh lemon juice and season with 1/4 tsp black pepper. Adjust salt and pepper to taste.
5. **Serve:** Divide the noodles into four bowls and top with optional sun-dried tomatoes, nutritional yeast, or red pepper flakes for added flavor.

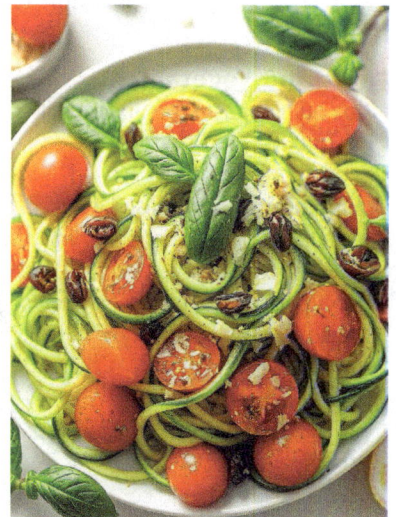

Nutritional Information (per serving)
- **Calories**: 120 kcal
- **Protein**: 3 g
- **Carbohydrates**: 12 g
- **Fats**: 7 g
- **Fiber**: 3 g
- **Cholesterol**: 0 mg
- **Sodium**: 170 mg
- **Potassium**: 450 mg

TURMERIC RICE NOODLES WITH VEGETABLES

Yield: 4 servings • Preparation Time: 15 minutes • Cooking Time: 10 minutes

Ingredients
Noodles and Vegetables
› **8 oz** rice noodles
› **1 tbsp** olive oil or avocado oil
› **1 medium red bell pepper**, thinly sliced
› **1 cup** broccoli florets
› **1 medium zucchini**, thinly sliced into half moons
› **1 medium carrot**, julienned or shredded
› **2 cups** baby spinach
Turmeric Sauce
› **1 tbsp** fresh ginger, grated
› **1 clove** garlic, minced
› **1 tsp** ground turmeric
› **1/2 tsp** ground cumin
› **1/2 tsp** ground coriander
› **2 tbsp** low-sodium tamari or soy sauce
› **1 tbsp** lime juice
› **1/2 cup** coconut milk (unsweetened)
Optional Add-Ins
› **1/4 tsp** red pepper flakes for heat
› **1 tbsp** sesame seeds or chia seeds for texture
› **1/4 cup** chopped fresh cilantro

Instructions
1. **Cook the Rice Noodles:** Bring a large pot of water to a boil, add 8 oz rice noodles, and cook according to package instructions, usually about 5–7 minutes, until tender. Drain, rinse under cold water, and set aside.
2. **Prepare the Turmeric Sauce:** In a small bowl, whisk together 1 tbsp grated ginger, 1 minced garlic clove, 1 tsp turmeric, 1/2 tsp cumin, 1/2 tsp coriander, 2 tbsp tamari, 1 tbsp lime juice, and 1/2 cup coconut milk until well combined. Set aside.
3. **Sauté the Vegetables:** In a large skillet or wok, heat 1 tbsp oil over medium heat. Add 1 sliced red bell pepper, 1 cup broccoli florets, 1 sliced zucchini, and 1 julienned carrot. Sauté for 4–5 minutes, until vegetables are tender-crisp but still vibrant.
4. **Add the Spinach and Sauce:** Add 2 cups baby spinach to the skillet and cook for another 1–2 minutes, just until wilted. Pour the turmeric sauce over the vegetables, stirring gently to coat.
5. **Combine Noodles with Sauce and Vegetables:** Add the cooked rice noodles to the skillet, tossing to coat them evenly in the sauce. Cook for an additional 1–2 minutes to heat through.
6. **Add Optional Garnishes:** For added texture and flavor, sprinkle with 1 tbsp sesame or chia seeds and garnish with 1/4 cup chopped fresh cilantro. Add 1/4 tsp red pepper flakes if you like a bit of heat.
7. **Serve:** Divide into four bowls and serve immediately. Enjoy warm.

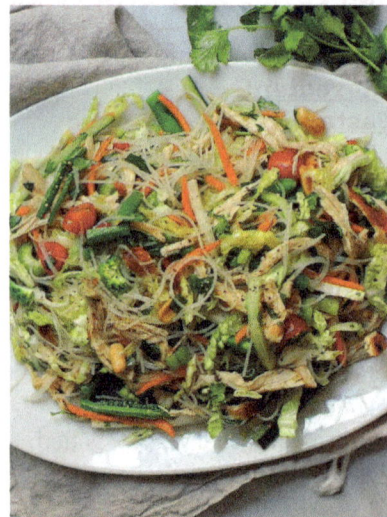

Nutritional Information (per serving)
- **Calories**: 280 kcal
- **Fiber**: 5 g
- **Protein**: 6 g
- **Cholesterol**: 0 mg
- **Carbohydrates**: 42 g
- **Sodium**: 280 mg
- **Fats**: 10 g
- **Potassium**: 520 mg

QUINOA PASTA PRIMAVERA WITH ARTICHOKE HEARTS

Yield: 4 servings • Preparation Time: 15 minutes • Cooking Time: 15 minutes

Ingredients
Pasta and Vegetables
› **8 oz** quinoa pasta (penne or fusilli)
› **1 tbsp** olive oil
› **1 cup** cherry tomatoes, halved
› **1 medium zucchini**, sliced into half moons
› **1/2 cup** yellow bell pepper, thinly sliced
› **1 cup** asparagus tips, cut into 1-inch pieces
› **1/2 cup** artichoke hearts (canned or jarred, rinsed and chopped)
› **1/4 tsp** sea salt
› **1/4 tsp** black pepper
Lemon Herb Dressing
› **3 tbsp** olive oil
› **2 tbsp** fresh lemon juice
› **1 clove** garlic, minced
› **1 tbsp** fresh basil, chopped
› **1 tbsp** fresh parsley, chopped
› **1 tsp** dried oregano
› **1/4 tsp** turmeric powder (for anti-inflammatory benefits)
› **1/4 tsp** crushed red pepper flakes (optional for a little heat)

Instructions
1. **Cook the Quinoa Pasta:** In a large pot, bring salted water to a boil. Add quinoa pasta and cook according to package instructions until al dente, typically 8–10 minutes. Drain and set aside.
2. **Sauté the Vegetables:** In a large skillet, heat 1 tbsp of olive oil over medium heat. Add cherry tomatoes, zucchini, yellow bell pepper, and asparagus tips. Sauté for 5–7 minutes until the vegetables are just tender but still vibrant in color. Season with sea salt and black pepper, then add the chopped artichoke hearts. Cook for an additional 2 min.
3. **Prepare the Lemon Herb Dressing:** In a small bowl, whisk together olive oil, lemon juice, minced garlic, fresh basil, parsley, dried oregano, turmeric powder, and crushed red pepper flakes. Stir well to combine.
4. **Combine Pasta and Vegetables:** In a large mixing bowl, combine the cooked quinoa pasta, sautéed vegetables, and artichoke hearts. Drizzle with the lemon herb dressing and toss gently to coat everything evenly.
5. **Serve:** Divide the pasta primavera into four servings. Serve warm or at room temperature.

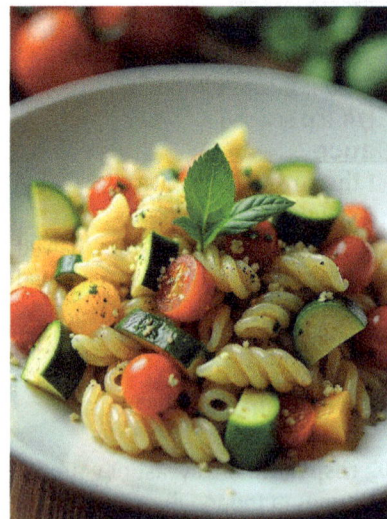

Nutritional Information (per serving)
- **Calories**: 320 kcal
- **Fiber**: 8 g
- **Protein**: 10 g
- **Cholesterol**: 0 mg
- **Carbohydrates**: 42 g
- **Sodium**: 200 mg
- **Fats**: 13 g
- **Potassium**: 550 mg

SPAGHETTI SQUASH WITH ROASTED GARLIC AND PARSLEY

Yield: 4 servings • Preparation Time: 15 minutes • Cooking Time: 45 minutes

Ingredients
> **1 large** spaghetti squash (about 2–3 pounds)
> **2 tbsp** extra virgin olive oil, divided
> **1 whole** garlic bulb
> **1/4 tsp** sea salt
> **1/4 tsp** black pepper
> **1/4 cup** fresh parsley, chopped
> **2 tbsp** lemon juice (about half a lemon)
> **1/4 tsp** crushed red pepper flakes (optional, for a bit of heat)

Optional Add-Ons
> **2 tbsp** toasted pine nuts or slivered almonds, for added crunch and healthy fats
> **1 tbsp** nutritional yeast, for a slightly cheesy flavor

Instructions
1. **Prepare and Roast the Spaghetti Squash:** Preheat your oven to 400°F (200°C). Carefully slice the spaghetti squash in half lengthwise and scoop out the seeds. Drizzle each half with 1 tablespoon of olive oil and sprinkle with sea salt and black pepper. Place the squash cut-side down on a baking sheet lined with parchment paper.
2. **Roast the Garlic:** Cut the top off the garlic bulb to expose the cloves, drizzle with a small amount of olive oil, and wrap it in foil. Place the wrapped garlic bulb on the baking sheet with the spaghetti squash. Roast everything for 35–45 minutes, until the squash is tender and the garlic is soft and golden.
3. **Shred the Squash:** Once the squash is cooked, use a fork to scrape the inside and create spaghetti-like strands. Transfer the strands to a large mixing bowl.
4. **Make the Roasted Garlic Sauce:** Carefully unwrap the garlic and squeeze the soft, roasted cloves into a small bowl. Mash the garlic cloves with a fork until smooth, then mix in the remaining olive oil, lemon juice, and chopped parsley.
5. **Combine and Season:** Pour the roasted garlic and parsley mixture over the spaghetti squash strands. Toss gently to combine. Sprinkle with crushed red pepper flakes if you'd like a little heat, and season with extra salt and pepper if needed.
6. **Serve:** Divide into four servings and top with optional pine nuts, slivered almonds, or a sprinkle of nutritional yeast for added flavor.

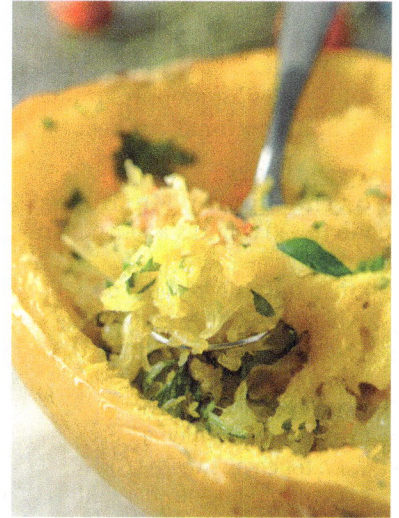

Nutritional Information (per serving)
- **Calories**: 145 kcal
- **Protein**: 2 g
- **Carbohydrates**: 18 g
- **Fats**: 8 g
- **Fiber**: 4 g
- **Cholesterol**: 0 mg
- **Sodium**: 150 mg
- **Potassium**: 420 mg

LENTIL PASTA WITH ROASTED TOMATO SAUCE

Yield: 4 servings • Preparation Time: 10 minutes • Cooking Time: 30 minutes (includes roasting time)

Ingredients

Roasted Tomato Sauce
> **2 cups** cherry or grape tomatoes, halved
> **1 tbsp** extra-virgin olive oil
> **4 cloves** garlic, unpeeled
> **1/4 tsp** sea salt
> **1/4 tsp** black pepper
> **1/2 tsp** dried oregano
> **1/4 tsp** red pepper flakes (optional, for a bit of heat)

Pasta
> **8 oz** lentil pasta (such as red or green lentil pasta)
> **1 tbsp** extra-virgin olive oil
> **1/4 cup** fresh basil, chopped
> **1 tbsp** nutritional yeast (optional, for a cheesy flavor and added nutrients)

Optional Add-ins
> **1/2 cup** sautéed mushrooms for extra flavor and nutrients
> **1/4 cup** chopped fresh parsley

Instructions
1. **Roast the Tomatoes and Garlic:** Preheat your oven to 400°F (200°C). On a baking sheet, spread the halved tomatoes and add the unpeeled garlic cloves. Drizzle with 1 tablespoon of olive oil, sprinkle with sea salt, black pepper, oregano, and optional red pepper flakes. Roast in the oven for 20–25 minutes, until tomatoes are softened and slightly caramelized.
2. **Cook the Lentil Pasta:** While the tomatoes are roasting, bring a large pot of water to a boil. Add the lentil pasta and cook according to package instructions, typically about 7–10 minutes. Drain and set aside.
3. **Prepare the Tomato Sauce:** Once the tomatoes are done roasting, remove the garlic cloves and peel them. In a blender or food processor, combine the roasted tomatoes, peeled garlic, and any remaining juices from the baking sheet. Blend until smooth for a creamy sauce, or pulse lightly if you prefer a chunkier texture.
4. **Combine Pasta and Sauce:** In a large skillet, heat 1 tablespoon of olive oil over medium heat. Add the cooked pasta and pour in the roasted tomato sauce. Toss to coat the pasta thoroughly in the sauce, and cook for an additional 2–3 minutes to heat through.
5. **Add Fresh Herbs and Nutritional Yeast:** Stir in fresh basil and nutritional yeast for a savory depth of flavor. Adjust seasoning as needed with additional salt or pepper.
6. **Serve:** Divide the pasta into bowls, garnish with more fresh basil, and add optional toppings for extra flavor.

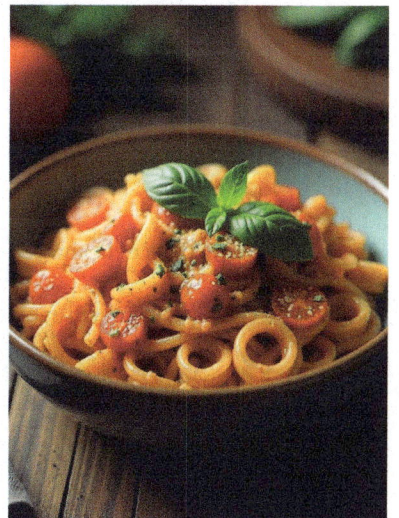

Nutritional Information (per serving)
- **Calories**: 330 kcal
- **Protein**: 15 g
- **Carbohydrates**: 45 g
- **Fats**: 10 g
- **Fiber**: 8 g
- **Cholesterol**: 0 mg
- **Sodium**: 250 mg
- **Potassium**: 600 mg

5. FISH AND SEAFOOD
LIGHT & FRESH

GINGER & LIME GRILLED SHRIMP SKEWERS

Yield: 4 servings (approximately 4 skewers per serving) • Preparation Time: 15 minutes • Marinating Time: 30 minutes to 1 hour (optional, for best flavor) • Cooking Time: 8–10 minutes

Ingredients
For the Shrimp Marinade:
> **1 lb** (16-20 count) shrimp, peeled and deveined
> **1 tbsp** fresh ginger, grated
> **2 tbsp** lime juice (freshly squeezed)
> **1 tbsp** olive oil
> **2 cloves** garlic, minced
> **1 tbsp** honey (optional, for a touch of sweetness)
> **1/2 tsp** turmeric powder (anti-inflammatory)
> **1/4 tsp** red pepper flakes
> **1/2 tsp** sea salt
> **1/4 tsp** black pepper

For the Grilling:
> **1 tbsp** olive oil (for brushing the grill or skewers)
> **Lime wedges**, for serving
> **Fresh cilantro**, chopped (for garnish)

Instructions
1. **Prepare the Shrimp Marinade:** In a medium bowl, combine the grated ginger, lime juice, olive oil, minced garlic, honey (if using), turmeric powder, red pepper flakes, sea salt, and black pepper. Stir well to combine into a marinade.
2. **Marinate the Shrimp:** Add the shrimp to the marinade and toss to coat evenly. Cover the bowl and refrigerate for 30 minutes to 1 hour, allowing the flavors to meld. If short on time, you can marinate for as little as 15 minutes.
3. **Prepare the Grill:** Preheat your grill to medium-high heat (about 375°F or 190°C). If using a grill pan, preheat it on the stove. Lightly brush the grill or skewers with olive oil to prevent the shrimp from sticking.
4. **Skewer the Shrimp:** Thread the marinated shrimp onto skewers (about 4-5 shrimp per skewer). If using wooden skewers, make sure to soak them in water for 10-15 minutes beforehand to prevent burning.
5. **Grill the Shrimp:** Place the skewers on the preheated grill. Grill the shrimp for 2-3 minutes per side, or until they are pink and opaque, with grill marks. Be careful not to overcook, as shrimp can become tough quickly.
6. **Serve:** Remove the shrimp from the skewers and transfer them to a serving platter. Garnish with freshly chopped cilantro and serve with lime wedges on the side.

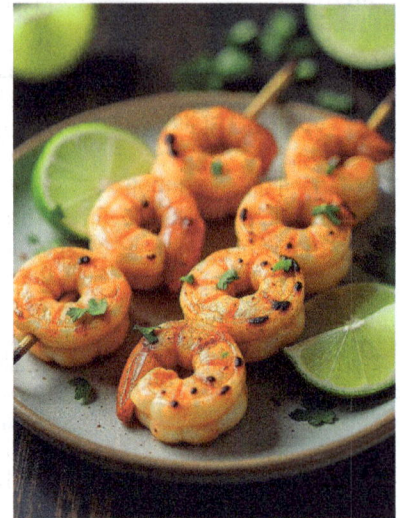

Nutritional Information (per serving, 1 skewer)
- **Calories**: 150 kcal
- **Protein**: 22 g
- **Carbohydrates**: 7 g
- **Fats**: 6 g
- **Fiber**: 1 g
- **Cholesterol**: 160 mg
- **Sodium**: 350 mg
- **Potassium**: 250 mg

LEMON-PEPPER BAKED COD WITH FRESH PARSLEY

Yield: 4 servings • Preparation Time: 10 minutes • Cooking Time: 15-20 minutes

Ingredients
For the Fish:
> **4 (6 oz)** cod fillets
> **1 tbsp** olive oil
> **1 tbsp** fresh lemon juice (from 1 lemon)
> **1 tsp** lemon zest (for extra citrus flavor)
> **1 tsp** black pepper
> **1/2 tsp** sea salt (or to taste)
> **1/2 tsp** garlic powder (optional, for added flavor)
> **1/2 tsp** smoked paprika (optional, adds depth and anti-inflammatory benefits)
> **1 tbsp** fresh parsley, chopped (for garnish)
> **Lemon wedges** (for serving)

Instructions
1. **Preheat the Oven** Preheat your oven to 400°F (200°C). Line a baking sheet with parchment paper or lightly grease it with olive oil to prevent the cod from sticking.
2. **Prepare the Cod Fillets:** Pat the cod fillets dry with paper towels to remove any excess moisture. This will help the fish bake properly and develop a slightly crispy exterior.
3. **Season the Cod:** Place the cod fillets on the prepared baking sheet. Drizzle the fillets with olive oil and fresh lemon juice. Sprinkle lemon zest, black pepper, sea salt, and garlic powder (if using) over the top. For additional flavor, sprinkle smoked paprika and turmeric (optional).
4. **Bake the Cod**: Bake the cod in the preheated oven for 15-20 minutes, or until the fish flakes easily with a fork. The exact time may vary depending on the thickness of your fillets, but the fish should reach an internal temperature of 145°F (63°C) when done.
5. **Garnish and Serve:** Once baked, remove the cod from the oven and transfer to serving plates. Garnish with freshly chopped parsley and serve with lemon wedges on the side.

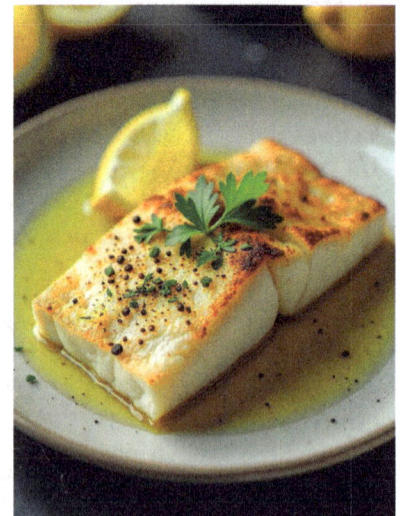

Nutritional Information (per serving)
- **Calories**: 230 kcal
- **Protein**: 28 g
- **Carbohydrates**: 2 g
- **Fats**: 12 g
- **Saturated fat**: 1.5 g
- **Monounsaturated fat**: 8 g
- **Fiber**: 1 g
- **Cholesterol**: 50 mg
- **Sodium**: 380 mg
- **Potassium**: 480 mg

CUCUMBER & DILL SALMON CEVICHE

Yield: 4 servings • Prep Time: 15 minutes • Passive Cooking (Marinating) Time: 30-45 minutes

Ingredients:

> **1 lb** fresh salmon fillet, skin removed, cut into 1/2-inch cubes
> **1/2 cup** fresh lime juice (about 4-5 limes)
> **1/2 medium** cucumber, diced
> **1/4** red onion, finely diced
> **1 small** avocado, diced
> **1/4 cup** fresh dill, finely chopped
> **1/4 cup** fresh cilantro, chopped
> **1 tbsp** extra-virgin olive oil
> **1/4 tsp** sea salt
> **1/4 tsp** black pepper
> **1/2 tsp** ground turmeric (optional, for added anti-inflammatory benefits)

Optional Toppings:

> Fresh dill sprigs or cilantro leaves
> **1 tbsp** pumpkin seeds (for added crunch and nutritional benefits)
> Slices of jalapeño (for a hint of heat)

Instructions:

1. **Prepare the Salmon:** Place the cubed salmon in a glass or ceramic bowl (avoid metal as it may react with the citrus).
2. **Add Citrus Juices:** Pour the lime and lemon juices over the salmon, ensuring that the salmon is fully submerged. The acid from the citrus will "cook" the salmon.
3. **Marinate the Salmon:** Cover the bowl with plastic wrap and refrigerate for 30-45 minutes, or until the salmon becomes opaque.
4. **Prepare the Vegetables and Herbs:** While the salmon is marinating, prepare the cucumber, red onion, and avocado. Chop the fresh dill and cilantro.
5. **Combine Ingredients:** After marinating, drain some of the excess citrus juice from the salmon, leaving a small amount to keep it moist. Add the cucumber, red onion, avocado, dill, and cilantro to the salmon.
6. **Season and Add Oil:** Drizzle the olive oil over the mixture, and season with sea salt, black pepper, and turmeric (if using). Gently toss to combine all ingredients, being careful not to mash the avocado.
7. **Serve:** Transfer the ceviche to serving bowls or small plates. Garnish with fresh dill or cilantro leaves, pumpkin seeds for added crunch, and optional jalapeño slices for a touch of heat.

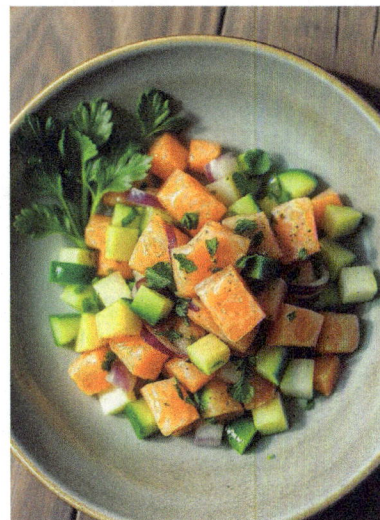

Nutritional Information (Per Serving):

- **Calories:** 250
- **Protein:** 20g
- **Carbohydrates:** 10g
- **Fats:** 15g
- **Fiber:** 4g
- **Cholesterol:** 40mg
- **Sodium:** 200mg
- **Potassium:** 600mg

STEAMED MUSSELS WITH GARLIC

Yield: 4 servings • Prep Time: 10 minutes • Cooking Time: 10 minutes

Ingredients:

> **2 lbs** fresh mussels, scrubbed and debearded
> **1 tbsp** extra-virgin olive oil
> **4 cloves** garlic, minced
> **1 small** shallot, finely chopped
> **1/2 cup** vegetable broth (or low-sodium chicken broth)
> **1/2 cup** white wine (optional; use broth as a substitute for non-alcoholic option)
> **1/2 tsp** ground turmeric
> **1/4 tsp** ground black pepper (to enhance turmeric absorption)
> **1 tbsp** fresh lemon juice
> **1/4 cup** fresh parsley, chopped
> **1/4 tsp** sea salt (optional, depending on sodium preference)
> **1/4 tsp** red pepper flakes (optional, for a hint of spice)

Optional Toppings:

> Additional chopped parsley for garnish
> Lemon wedges for serving
> **1 tbsp** pumpkin seeds (for added crunch and nutrients)

Instructions:

1. **Prepare the Mussels:** Rinse the mussels thoroughly under cold water, scrubbing the shells and removing any "beards" (the stringy fibers). Discard any mussels that remain open after tapping, as these may be spoiled.
2. **Heat the Olive Oil:** In a large, deep skillet or Dutch oven, heat the olive oil over medium heat.
3. **Sauté Garlic and Shallot:** Add the minced garlic and chopped shallot to the skillet. Sauté for 1-2 minutes, stirring frequently, until they are softened and fragrant, but not browned.
4. **Add Turmeric and Broth:** Sprinkle in the turmeric and black pepper, stirring well to combine and release their flavors. Pour in the vegetable broth and white wine (if using), and bring the mixture to a simmer.
5. **Steam the Mussels:** Add the mussels to the skillet, cover with a lid, and steam for 5-7 minutes, or until the mussels open fully. Shake the skillet gently a few times during cooking to ensure even steaming. Discard any mussels that do not open.
6. **Add Lemon Juice and Parsley:** Once the mussels are fully cooked, remove from heat. Stir in the lemon juice and chopped parsley, and season with sea salt and red pepper flakes if desired.
7. **Serve:** Transfer the mussels to serving bowls, pouring the remaining broth over the top. Garnish with additional parsley, a sprinkle of pumpkin seeds (if using), and lemon wedges on the side.

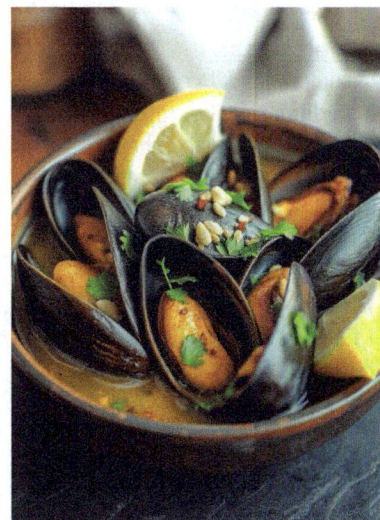

Nutritional Information (Per Serving):

- **Calories:** 220
- **Protein:** 23g
- **Carbohydrates:** 7g
- **Fats:** 10g
- **Fiber:** 1g
- **Cholesterol:** 45mg
- **Sodium:** 540mg
- **Potassium:** 490mg

MISO-MARINATED SEA BASS WITH BOK CHOY

Yield: 4 servings • Prep Time: 15 minutes • Passive Marinating Time: 30 minutes • Cooking Time: 15 minutes

Ingredients:

> **4** sea bass fillets (4 oz each)
> **3 tbsp** white miso paste
> **2 tbsp** rice vinegar
> **1 tbsp** fresh ginger, grated
> **1 tbsp** honey or maple syrup
> **1 tbsp** sesame oil (for added flavor and anti-inflammatory benefits)
> **1 tbsp** water (if needed, to thin the marinade)
> **1 tbsp** olive oil or avocado oil
> **4 cups** bok choy, halved lengthwise
> **1/4 tsp** sea salt
> **1/4 tsp** black pepper
> **1 tbsp** toasted sesame seeds (optional, for garnish)

Optional Toppings:

> Thinly sliced green onions
> Extra toasted sesame seeds
> Lime wedges for serving

Instructions:

1. **Prepare the Marinade:** In a small bowl, whisk together the miso paste, rice vinegar, grated ginger, honey, and sesame oil until smooth. If the mixture is too thick, add a bit of water to thin it to a spreadable consistency.
2. **Marinate the Sea Bass:** Pat the sea bass fillets dry with paper towels. Place them in a shallow dish and brush the miso marinade over each fillet, coating them evenly. Cover and marinate in the refrigerator for at least 30 minutes for optimal flavor.
3. **Preheat the Oven:** Preheat the oven to 400°F (200°C). Line a baking sheet with parchment paper or lightly oil it to prevent sticking.
4. **Cook the Bok Choy:** While the oven preheats, heat the olive oil in a large skillet over medium heat. Add the bok choy, cut side down, and season with sea salt and black pepper. Sauté for 3-4 minutes, or until slightly wilted and tender. Set aside.
5. **Bake the Sea Bass:** Place the marinated sea bass fillets on the prepared baking sheet. Bake in the preheated oven for 10-12 minutes, or until the fish is opaque and flakes easily with a fork.
6. **Serve:** Plate the baked sea bass alongside the sautéed bok choy. Sprinkle toasted sesame seeds and thinly sliced green onions over the top for garnish. Serve with lime wedges for a fresh citrus touch.

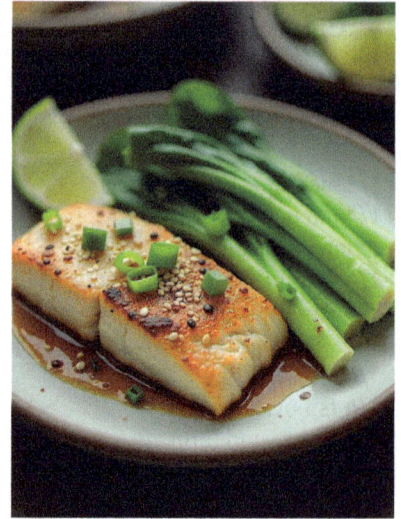

Nutritional Information (Per Serving):

- **Calories:** 220
- **Protein:** 20g
- **Carbohydrates:** 7g
- **Fats:** 12g
- **Fiber:** 2g
- **Cholesterol:** 45mg
- **Sodium:** 410mg
- **Potassium:** 500mg

HEARTIER FISH DISHES

BAKED SALMON WITH SWEET POTATO & FENNEL

Yield: 4 servings • Prep Time: 15 minutes • Cooking Time: 30 minutes

Ingredients:

> **4** salmon fillets (4 oz each)
> **2 medium** sweet potatoes, peeled and cut into 1-inch cubes
> **1** fennel bulb, thinly sliced (reserve fronds for garnish)
> **2 tbsp** olive oil, divided
> **1 tbsp** fresh lemon juice
> **1 tsp** lemon zest
> **1 tsp** fresh rosemary, chopped (or **1/2 tsp** dried rosemary)
> **1/2 tsp** sea salt (optional)
> **1/4 tsp** black pepper
> **1/2 tsp** turmeric powder (optional, for added anti-inflammatory benefit)
> **1 clove** garlic, minced

Optional Toppings:

> Chopped fennel fronds for garnish
> Fresh parsley, chopped
> Extra lemon wedges for serving

Instructions:

1. **Preheat the Oven:** Preheat your oven to 400°F (200°C). Line a baking sheet with parchment paper for easy cleanup.
2. **Prepare the Vegetables:** In a large bowl, toss the sweet potato cubes and fennel slices with 1 tablespoon of olive oil, rosemary, sea salt, black pepper, and turmeric powder (if using). Spread the seasoned vegetables evenly on the prepared baking sheet, keeping them on one side to leave space for the salmon.
3. **Bake the Vegetables:** Place the baking sheet in the oven and bake the vegetables for 15 minutes.
4. **Prepare the Salmon:** While the vegetables are baking, season the salmon fillets with lemon zest, lemon juice, garlic, and the remaining tablespoon of olive oil. Rub the seasoning onto each fillet to evenly coat the fish.
5. **Add Salmon to the Baking Sheet:** After 15 minutes, remove the baking sheet from the oven and place the seasoned salmon fillets on the empty side. Return the baking sheet to the oven and bake for another 12-15 minutes, or until the salmon is opaque and flakes easily with a fork, and the vegetables are tender.
6. **Serve:** Divide the salmon and roasted vegetables onto plates. Garnish with chopped fennel fronds and fresh parsley for added color and flavor. Serve with extra lemon wedges if desired.

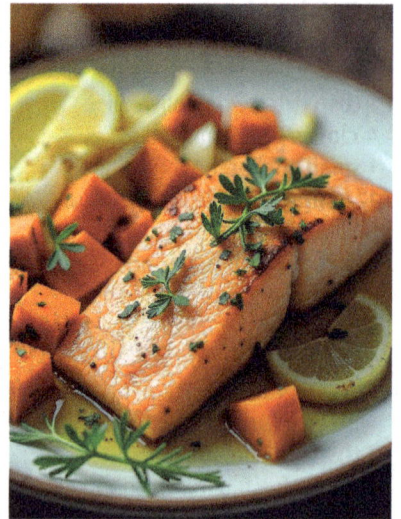

Nutritional Information (Per Serving):

- **Calories:** 350
- **Protein:** 28g
- **Carbohydrates:** 25g
- **Fats:** 16g
- **Fiber:** 6g
- **Cholesterol:** 60mg
- **Sodium:** 250mg
- **Potassium:** 900mg

MOROCCAN-SPICED FISH STEW WITH SAFFRON

Yield: 4 servings • Prep Time: 15 minutes • Cooking Time: 30 minutes

Ingredients:
> **1 lb** white fish fillets (such as cod or halibut), cut into 2-inch chunks
> **1 tbsp** olive oil
> **1 medium** onion, diced
> **2 cloves** garlic, minced
> **1-inch** piece fresh ginger, grated (or 1/2 tsp ground ginger)
> **1 tsp** ground turmeric
> **1 tsp** ground cumin
> **1/2 tsp** ground cinnamon
> **1/4 tsp** ground coriander
> **1 pinch** saffron threads (optional, for added flavor and nutrition)
> **1** red bell pepper, diced
> **1 medium** zucchini, diced
> **1 can** (14 oz) diced tomatoes, no salt added
> **2 cups** low-sodium vegetable broth or fish stock
> Salt and black pepper, to taste
> **1/4 cup** fresh cilantro, chopped (for garnish)
> **1/2** lemon, juiced (for garnish)

Optional Add-ins:
> **1/2 tsp** crushed red pepper flakes (for a bit of heat)
> **1/4 cup** sliced green olives (for an additional Moroccan touch)
> Fresh parsley, chopped (for garnish)

Instructions:
1. **Prepare the Saffron (Optional):** If using saffron, place the threads in a small bowl with 2 tablespoons of warm water. Let it steep while you prepare the stew to bring out its full flavor.
2. **Sauté the Aromatics:** Heat the olive oil in a large pot over medium heat. Add the diced onion and cook for about 5 minutes, until softened. Add the minced garlic and grated ginger, and cook for another minute, stirring constantly to prevent burning.
3. **Add the Spices:** Stir in the turmeric, cumin, cinnamon, coriander, and saffron (along with its soaking liquid, if used). Let the spices toast for 1-2 minutes to release their aroma.
4. **Add the Vegetables:** Add the diced red bell pepper, zucchini, and diced tomatoes (with their juices) to the pot. Stir to combine the vegetables with the spices.
5. **Simmer the Stew:** Pour in the vegetable broth or fish stock, season with salt and pepper to taste, and bring the mixture to a simmer. Let it cook for 15-20 minutes, allowing the flavors to meld and the vegetables to soften.
6. **Add the Fish:** Gently add the fish chunks to the stew, making sure they are mostly submerged in the broth. Let the fish simmer for 5-7 minutes, or until it is opaque and flakes easily with a fork.
7. **Finish with Lemon and Garnish:** Once the fish is cooked, remove the pot from heat and stir in the lemon juice. Garnish with fresh cilantro and any additional parsley or green olives, if desired.

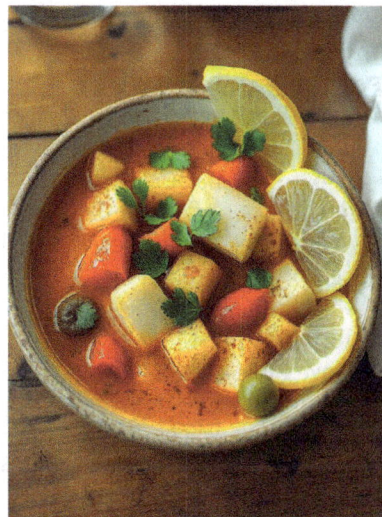

Nutritional Information (Per Serving):
- **Calories:** 240
- **Protein:** 28g
- **Carbohydrates:** 15g
- **Fats:** 8g
- **Fiber:** 5g
- **Cholesterol:** 60mg
- **Sodium:** 380mg
- **Potassium:** 750mg

BROILED TUNA STEAKS WITH MANGO SALSA

Yield: 4 servings • Prep Time: 15 minutes • Cooking Time: 8-10 minutes • Setting Time: 5 minutes (for resting after broiling)

Ingredients:
Tuna Steaks
> **4** tuna steaks (5 oz each, about 1-inch thick)
> **1 tbsp** olive oil
> **1 tbsp** fresh lime juice
> **1/2 tsp** ground black pepper
> **1/4 tsp** sea salt (optional)
> **1/2 tsp** ground cumin

Mango Salsa
> **1** ripe mango, diced
> **1/2 small** red onion, finely diced
> **1/2** red bell pepper, finely diced
> **1/2** jalapeño, finely diced (optional for spice)
> **1/4 cup** fresh cilantro, chopped
> Juice of 1 lime
> **1/4 tsp** ground turmeric (optional, for anti-inflammatory boost)

Instructions:
1. **Prepare the Tuna Steaks:** Pat the tuna steaks dry with paper towels to remove excess moisture. This will help them sear well under the broiler. In a small bowl, mix together the olive oil, lime juice, ground black pepper, sea salt, and cumin. Brush the marinade evenly over each side of the tuna steaks, and let them sit for a few minutes to absorb the flavors while you prepare the salsa.
2. **Prepare the Mango Salsa:** In a medium bowl, combine the diced mango, red onion, red bell pepper, jalapeño (if using), fresh cilantro, lime juice, and turmeric (if using). Gently toss the ingredients together until evenly mixed. Set aside to allow the flavors to meld while you cook the tuna.
3. **Broil the Tuna:** Preheat the broiler on high and adjust the oven rack so that it is about 4 inches from the broiler. Line a baking sheet with foil and place the marinated tuna steaks on the sheet. Broil the tuna for 4-5 minutes on each side, or until it reaches your desired doneness. (For medium-rare, cook until the tuna is just opaque and still slightly pink in the center.)
4. **Rest and Serve:** Remove the tuna from the broiler and allow it to rest for 5 minutes to let the juices redistribute. Spoon a generous amount of mango salsa over each tuna steak. Garnish with additional fresh cilantro if desired.

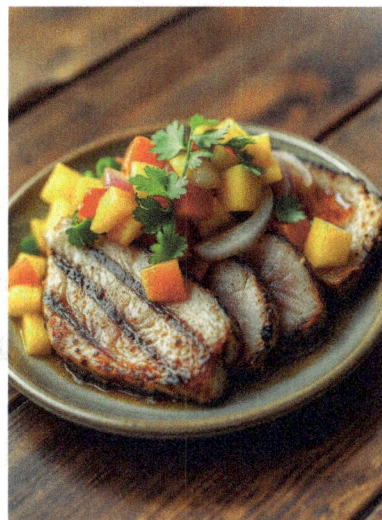

Nutritional Information (Per Serving):
- **Calories:** 295
- **Protein:** 34g
- **Carbohydrates:** 15g
- **Fats:** 11g
- **Fiber:** 3g
- **Cholesterol:** 45mg
- **Sodium:** 210mg
- **Potassium:** 750mg

SALMON & SPINACH PATTIES WITH LEMON-DILL SAUCE

Yield: 4 servings (8 patties) • Prep Time: 15 minutes • Cook Time: 10 minutes • Passive Time: 10 minutes chilling (optional, for easier handling)

Ingredients:
For the Salmon Patties:
> **1 lb** fresh or canned salmon, drained and flaked
> **1 cup** fresh spinach, chopped
> **1/4 cup** almond flour (or oat flour)
> **1/4 cup** green onion, finely chopped
> **1 egg**, beaten
> **1 tbsp** fresh dill, chopped
> **1 tbsp** lemon zest
> **1 clove** garlic, minced
> **1/4 tsp** sea salt
> **1/4 tsp** black pepper
> **1 tbsp** olive oil or avocado oil (for cooking)

For the Lemon-Dill Sauce:
> **1/2 cup** plain Greek yogurt (or dairy-free yogurt if preferred)
> **1 tbsp** fresh lemon juice
> **1 tbsp** fresh dill, chopped
> Salt and pepper to taste

Optional Additions:
> **1/2 tsp** smoked paprika or cumin for added flavor
> **1/4 cup** finely grated zucchini for extra moisture

Instructions:
1. **Prepare the Salmon Mixture:** In a medium bowl, combine the flaked salmon, chopped spinach, almond flour, green onion, beaten egg, fresh dill, lemon zest, garlic, salt, and pepper. Mix until all ingredients are well-incorporated. If the mixture feels too soft, chill it in the fridge for about 10 minutes to help it firm up.
2. **Form the Patties:** Using your hands, shape the salmon mixture into 8 small patties (about 2 inches wide). Press gently to ensure they hold together.
3. **Cook the Patties:** Heat the olive or avocado oil in a non-stick skillet over medium heat. Add the salmon patties in a single layer (cook in batches if necessary to avoid overcrowding). Cook for 3-4 minutes on each side, or until golden brown and cooked through. Be careful when flipping to keep them intact.
4. **Prepare the Lemon-Dill Sauce:** In a small bowl, combine the Greek yogurt, lemon juice, fresh dill, and a pinch of salt and pepper. Stir until smooth.
5. **Serve:** Place the cooked patties on a serving plate and drizzle or serve with the Lemon-Dill Sauce on the side.

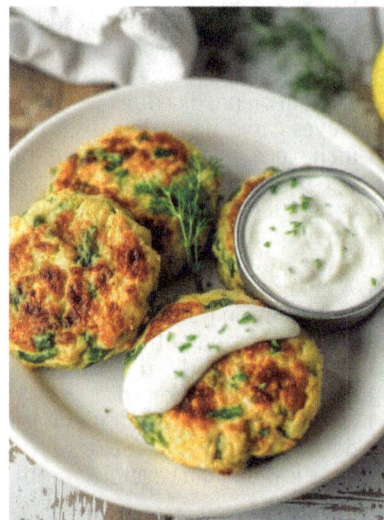

Nutritional Information (Per Serving):
- **Calories:** 230
- **Protein:** 23g
- **Carbohydrates:** 4g
- **Fats:** 14g
- **Fiber:** 1g
- **Cholesterol:** 70mg
- **Sodium:** 280mg
- **Potassium:** 540mg

GRILLED SWORDFISH WITH OLIVE & TOMATO RELISH

Yield: 4 servings • Prep Time: 15 minutes • Cook Time: 10 minutes • Passive Time: 10 minutes (for marinating)

Ingredients:
For the Swordfish:
> **4** swordfish steaks (about 4-5 oz each)
> **2 tbsp** olive oil
> **1 tbsp** fresh lemon juice
> **1 clove** garlic, minced
> **1/2 tsp** sea salt
> **1/4 tsp** black pepper
> **1/2 tsp** smoked paprika (optional for a smoky flavor)

For the Olive & Tomato Relish:
> **1 cup** cherry tomatoes, halved
> **1/2 cup** Kalamata olives, pitted and roughly chopped
> **1/4 cup** red onion, finely chopped
> **1 tbsp** fresh basil, chopped
> **1 tbsp** fresh parsley, chopped
> **1 tbsp** capers, drained
> **1 tbsp** extra-virgin olive oil
> **1 tbsp** balsamic vinegar
> Salt and pepper to taste

Instructions:
1. **Prepare the Swordfish Marinade:** In a small bowl, mix the olive oil, lemon juice, minced garlic, sea salt, black pepper, and smoked paprika (if using). Place the swordfish steaks in a shallow dish and pour the marinade over them. Allow the fish to marinate for about 10 minutes.
2. **Preheat the Grill:** Preheat your grill or grill pan to medium-high heat (around 400°F).
3. **Prepare the Olive & Tomato Relish:** In a medium bowl, combine the halved cherry tomatoes, Kalamata olives, red onion, basil, parsley, and capers. Drizzle with extra-virgin olive oil and balsamic vinegar, then season with a pinch of salt and pepper. Toss to combine and set aside.
4. **Grill the Swordfish:** Once the grill is hot, place the marinated swordfish steaks on the grill. Grill for about 4-5 minutes per side, or until the fish reaches an internal temperature of 145°F and is opaque. Remove from the grill and let the swordfish rest for a few minutes.
5. **Serve:** Plate the grilled swordfish and spoon the olive & tomato relish generously over the top. Garnish with extra fresh herbs if desired.

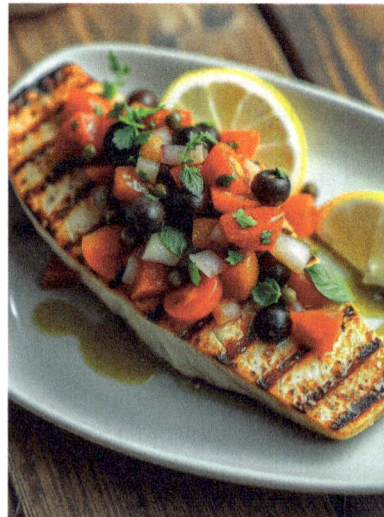

Nutritional Information (Per Serving):
- **Calories:** 320
- **Protein:** 35g
- **Carbohydrates:** 5g
- **Fats:** 18g
- **Fiber:** 2g
- **Cholesterol:** 85mg
- **Sodium:** 590mg
- **Potassium:** 700mg

WHITE FISH & SWEET POTATO COCONUT STEW

Yield: 4 servings • Prep Time: 15 minutes • Cook Time: 30 minutes • Passive Time: None

Ingredients:

> 1 **lb (450g)** white fish fillets (such as cod, haddock, or tilapia), cut into 2-inch pieces
> 1 **tbsp** coconut oil or olive oil
> 1 **medium** onion, finely chopped
> 3 **cloves** garlic, minced
> 1 **tbsp** fresh ginger, grated
> 1/2 **tsp** ground turmeric
> 1/2 **tsp** ground cumin
> 1/4 **tsp** ground coriander (optional)
> 1 **medium** sweet potato, peeled and cut into 1/2-inch cubes (about 1.5 cups)
> 1 red bell pepper, diced
> 1 **can** (14 oz) coconut milk (full-fat for a creamier stew)
> 1 **cup** low-sodium vegetable broth or water
> 1 **tbsp** fresh lime juice
> Sea salt and black pepper, to taste
> 1/4 **cup** fresh cilantro, chopped (for garnish)
> 1/4 **cup** scallions, sliced (for garnish)

Optional Ingredients:

> 1/2 **tsp** chili flakes or a small pinch of cayenne for heat
> 1 **cup** baby spinach or kale leaves for added greens

Instructions:

1. **Sauté the Aromatics:** Heat the coconut oil in a large pot or Dutch oven over medium heat. Add the chopped onion and cook until softened, about 3-4 minutes. Add the garlic and ginger, cooking for an additional minute until fragrant.
2. **Add the Spices:** Stir in the turmeric, cumin, and coriander (if using). Let the spices cook with the aromatics for 1-2 minutes, enhancing their flavors.
3. **Add the Sweet Potato and Red Pepper:** Add the diced sweet potato and red bell pepper to the pot, stirring to coat them with the spices. Cook for another 2-3 minutes.
4. **Pour in the Coconut Milk and Broth:** Add the coconut milk and vegetable broth, stirring to combine. Bring the mixture to a gentle boil, then reduce the heat to low. Cover and simmer for 15-20 minutes, or until the sweet potato is tender.
5. **Add the Fish:** Gently add the pieces of white fish to the stew, submerging them in the liquid. Cover and simmer for an additional 5-7 minutes, or until the fish is cooked through and flakes easily with a fork.
6. **Season and Add Lime Juice:** Stir in the fresh lime juice and season with salt and black pepper to taste. Add chili flakes or cayenne if you'd like a bit of heat. If adding greens like spinach or kale, stir them in and cook until just wilted.
7. **Garnish and Serve:** Ladle the stew into bowls and garnish with fresh cilantro and scallions. Serve warm.

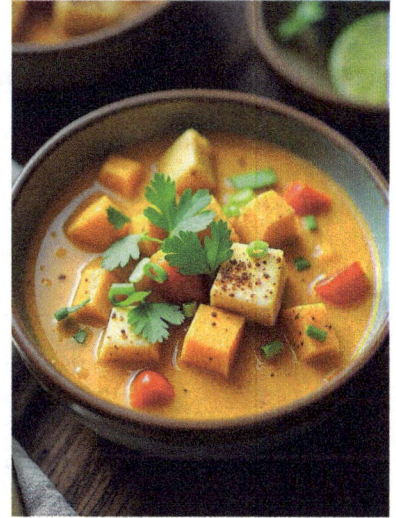

Nutritional Information (Per Serving):

- **Calories:** 360
- **Protein:** 28g
- **Carbohydrates:** 20g
- **Fats:** 20g
- **Fiber:** 4g
- **Cholesterol:** 50mg
- **Sodium:** 400mg
- **Potassium:** 870mg

6. POULTRY RECIPES
LIGHTER POULTRY RECIPES

LEMON & HERB CHICKEN SKEWERS WITH CUCUMBER SALAD

Yield: 4 servings • Prep Time: 15 minutes • Cook Time: 10-12 minutes • Passive Time: 15-30 minutes (for marination)

Ingredients:
For the Chicken Skewers:

> 1 **lb (450g)** boneless, skinless chicken breast, cut into 1.5-inch cubes
> 2 **tbsp** extra-virgin olive oil
> Zest and juice of 1 lemon
> 2 **garlic cloves**, minced
> 1 **tbsp** fresh oregano, chopped (or 1 tsp dried oregano)
> 1 **tbsp** fresh thyme, chopped (or 1 tsp dried thyme)
> 1/2 **tsp** ground turmeric
> 1/4 **tsp** ground black pepper
> 1/2 **tsp** sea salt (or to taste)
> 1 **tbsp** fresh parsley, chopped (for garnish)

For the Cucumber Salad:

> 1 **large** cucumber, thinly sliced
> 1/4 red onion, thinly sliced
> 1 **tbsp** fresh dill, chopped
> 1 **tbsp** extra-virgin olive oil
> 1 **tbsp** apple cider vinegar
> 1/2 **tsp** sea salt (or to taste)
> Freshly cracked black pepper, to taste
> 1 **tbsp** fresh lemon juice (optional for extra tang)

Optional:

> Cherry tomatoes or bell peppers, chopped (for added color and flavor)
> A sprinkle of sesame seeds for extra crunch

Instructions:

1. **Marinate the Chicken:** In a bowl, combine the olive oil, lemon zest, lemon juice, minced garlic, oregano, thyme, turmeric, black pepper, and salt. Stir well to create the marinade. Add the chicken pieces to the marinade, tossing to coat evenly. Cover and refrigerate for at least 15-30 minutes to allow the flavors to infuse (overnight marination will intensify the flavors).
2. **Prepare the Cucumber Salad:** In a separate bowl, combine the cucumber slices, red onion, and fresh dill. Drizzle with olive oil, apple cider vinegar, salt, and pepper. Toss gently to mix, then set aside to marinate for a few minutes. If you like extra tang, add lemon juice. Optionally, toss in some cherry tomatoes or bell peppers for added flavor and color. Allow the salad to sit while you cook the chicken so the flavors can develop.
3. **Assemble the Skewers:** Preheat the grill or grill pan over medium-high heat. If using wooden skewers, soak them in water for 10-15 minutes to prevent burning. Thread the marinated chicken pieces onto the skewers, leaving a small gap between each piece for even cooking.
4. **4Grill the Chicken Skewers:** Place the skewers on the preheated grill. Cook for 4-5 minutes on each side, or until the chicken is cooked through and the internal temperature reaches 165°F (74°C). Optionally, squeeze fresh lemon juice over the chicken skewers before serving for extra flavor.
5. **Serve:** Serve the chicken skewers with the cucumber salad on the side. Garnish the skewers with freshly chopped parsley for a pop of color and flavor.

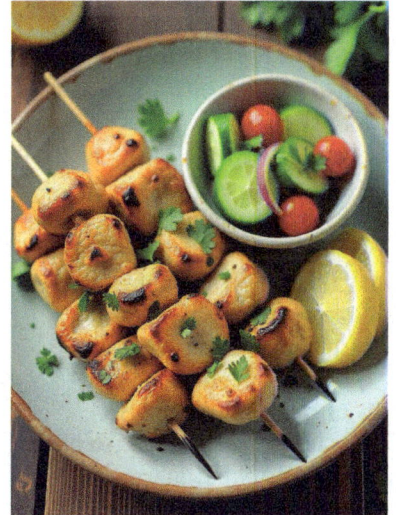

Nutritional Information (Per Serving):

- **Calories:** 290
- **Protein:** 32g
- **Carbohydrates:** 10g
- **Fats:** 14g
- **Fiber:** 3g
- **Cholesterol:** 70mg
- **Sodium:** 470mg
- **Potassium:** 800mg

CILANTRO-GINGER MARINATED CHICKEN BREAST

Yield: 4 servings • Prep Time: 10 minutes • Cook Time: 15-20 minutes • Passive Time (for marinating): 30 minutes to 2 hours

Ingredients:
For the Chicken Marinade:
› **1 lb** (450g) boneless, skinless chicken breasts
› **2 tbsp** fresh cilantro, finely chopped (plus extra for garnish)
› **1 tbsp** fresh ginger, grated
› **2 garlic cloves**, minced
› **2 tbsp** olive oil (extra virgin)
› **1 tbsp** apple cider vinegar
› Zest and juice of 1 lime
› **1 tbsp** honey (optional for a touch of sweetness)
› **1 tsp** ground turmeric
› **1/2 tsp** ground cumin
› **1/2 tsp** sea salt (or to taste)
› **1/4 tsp** freshly ground black pepper

Optional Toppings:
› Sliced avocado
› Lime wedges
› Fresh parsley for garnish
› Sliced red chili for heat (optional)

Instructions:
1. **Prepare the Marinade:** In a bowl, combine the chopped cilantro, grated ginger, minced garlic, olive oil, apple cider vinegar, lime zest, lime juice, honey (if using), turmeric, cumin, salt, and black pepper. Mix well until the marinade is evenly combined.
2. **Marinate the Chicken:** Place the chicken breasts in a resealable plastic bag or shallow dish. Pour the marinade over the chicken, ensuring it is evenly coated. Seal the bag or cover the dish and refrigerate for at least 30 minutes, ideally 2 hours, to allow the flavors to infuse the chicken. (Marinating longer will intensify the flavor.)
3. **Cook the Chicken:** Preheat a grill or grill pan over medium heat. If using a regular pan, heat 1 tablespoon of olive oil over medium heat. Remove the chicken from the marinade, letting any excess marinade drip off. Grill or cook the chicken for about 7-8 minutes per side, or until the internal temperature reaches 165°F (74°C) and the juices run clear. If using a pan, you can also cook the chicken breasts by searing them for 3-4 minutes per side and then finishing in the oven at 375°F (190°C) for 5-10 minutes.
4. **Serve:** Once cooked, remove the chicken from the heat and let it rest for a few minutes. Slice the chicken and garnish with additional chopped cilantro. Optional: Serve with lime wedges, sliced avocado, or a sprinkle of fresh parsley for extra flavor and color.

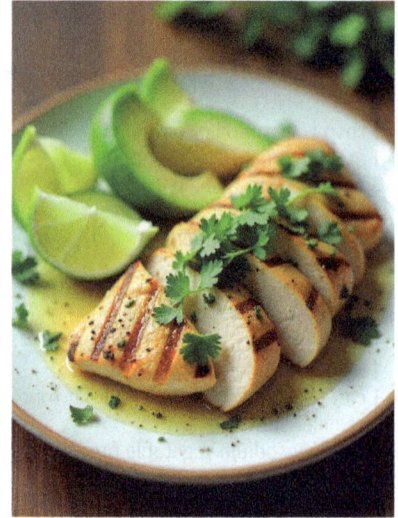

Nutritional Information (Per Serving):
- **Calories:** 250
- **Protein:** 38g
- **Carbohydrates:** 6g
- **Fats:** 10g
- **Fiber:** 2g
- **Cholesterol:** 70mg
- **Sodium:** 470mg
- **Potassium:** 720mg

ROASTED TURKEY BREAST WITH FRESH HERBS

Yield: 6 servings • Prep Time: 10 minutes • Cook Time: 1 hour 30 minutes • Rest Time: 10 minutes • Total Time: 1 hour 50 min.

Ingredients:
For the Roasted Turkey:
› **3 to 4 lbs** (1.4 to 1.8 kg) skinless, boneless turkey breast
› **2 tbsp** olive oil (extra virgin)
› **1 tbsp** fresh rosemary, finely chopped (or 1 tsp dried)
› **1 tbsp** fresh thyme, finely chopped (or 1 tsp dried)
› **1 tbsp** fresh sage, finely chopped (optional, for added flavor)
› **4 garlic cloves**, minced
› Zest of 1 lemon
› **1 tsp** ground turmeric
› **1/2 tsp** ground black pepper
› **1/2 tsp** sea salt (or to taste)
› **1/2 cup** low-sodium chicken broth (optional, for basting)

Optional Toppings:
› Fresh lemon wedges
› Fresh parsley, chopped (for garnish)
› Sautéed spinach or roasted vegetables on the side for additional anti-inflammatory benefits

Instructions:
1. **Prepare the Turkey:** Preheat the oven to 375°F (190°C). Pat the turkey breast dry with paper towels. This helps the seasoning adhere better and ensures crispy skin if you have skin on your turkey. Place the turkey breast on a large baking sheet or in a roasting pan.
2. **Make the Herb Marinade:** In a small bowl, combine the olive oil, minced garlic, fresh rosemary, thyme, sage (if using), lemon zest, ground turmeric, black pepper, and sea salt. Mix the ingredients well to form a paste-like marinade.
3. **Marinate the Turkey:** Rub the herb mixture all over the turkey breast, making sure to cover the entire surface. You can also gently lift the skin (if present) and rub the mixture underneath for extra flavor. Let the turkey sit for about 10 minutes to allow the flavors to meld. For a more intense flavor, you can refrigerate the turkey and let it marinate for up to 2 hours (or overnight).
4. **Roast the Turkey:** Place the turkey in the preheated oven and roast for 1 hour to 1 hour and 30 minutes, depending on the size of the breast. The turkey is done when the internal temperature reaches 165°F (74°C) in the thickest part of the breast. Optional: Halfway through roasting, baste the turkey with low-sodium chicken broth to keep it moist. If you don't want to use broth, you can baste with the pan juices.
5. **Rest and Slice:** Once cooked, remove the turkey from the oven and let it rest for 10 minutes before slicing. This helps the juices redistribute, making the turkey moist and tender.
6. **Serve:** Slice the turkey breast into even slices and arrange on a platter. Optional: Garnish with fresh parsley and serve with lemon wedges on the side for added brightness.

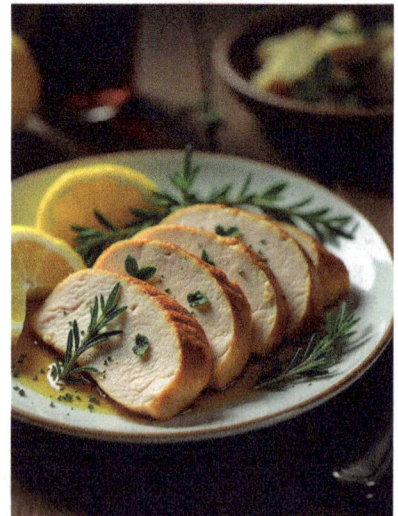

Nutritional Information (Per Serving):
- **Calories:** 280
- **Protein:** 50g
- **Carbohydrates:** 3g
- **Fats:** 10g
- **Fiber:** 1g
- **Cholesterol:** 90mg
- **Sodium:** 380mg
- **Potassium:** 540mg

TURMERIC CHICKEN TENDERS

Yield: 4 servings • Prep Time: 15 minutes • Cook Time: 20 minutes • Total Time: 35 minutes

Ingredients:
For the Chicken Tenders:
> **1 lb** (450g) boneless, skinless chicken tenders
> **2 tbsp** olive oil (extra virgin)
> **1 tbsp** turmeric powder
> **1 tsp** ground black pepper
> **1 tsp** garlic powder
> **1/2 tsp** ground ginger
> **1/2 tsp** paprika (for color and subtle smokiness)
> **1/2 tsp** sea salt (or to taste)
> **1 tbsp** lemon juice
> **1 tbsp** fresh cilantro, chopped (optional, for garnish)

Optional Dipping Sauce (Anti-Inflammatory Yogurt Sauce):
> **1/2 cup** plain Greek yogurt
> **1 tbsp** fresh lemon juice
> **1 tsp** ground turmeric
> **1/2 tsp** ground black pepper
> **1/2 tsp** honey (optional, for slight sweetness)
> **1 tbsp** fresh parsley, chopped (optional, for extra flavor)

Instructions:
1. **Prepare the Chicken:** Preheat your oven to 400°F (200°C). Line a baking sheet with parchment paper or lightly grease it with olive oil to prevent sticking. In a large bowl, combine olive oil, turmeric powder, black pepper, garlic powder, ground ginger, paprika, and sea salt. Stir well to create a marinade.
2. **Marinate the Chicken:** Add the chicken tenders to the bowl with the marinade. Toss well to ensure that the chicken is evenly coated in the spice mixture. Let it marinate for 10–15 minutes. If you have more time, you can marinate for up to 1 hour for more intense flavor.
3. **Cook the Chicken Tenders:** Once the chicken is marinated, place the tenders on the prepared baking sheet in a single layer. Roast the chicken in the preheated oven for 15–20 minutes, or until the chicken is cooked through and reaches an internal temperature of 165°F (74°C). Flip the chicken halfway through cooking for even browning.
4. **Optional Dipping Sauce:** While the chicken is cooking, prepare the dipping sauce by mixing together Greek yogurt, lemon juice, ground turmeric, black pepper, honey, and fresh parsley (if using) in a small bowl. Stir well to combine and refrigerate until ready to serve.
5. **Serve:** Once the chicken tenders are cooked, remove them from the oven and let them rest for 5 minutes. Serve the chicken tenders with the optional yogurt dipping sauce, and garnish with chopped cilantro for a fresh touch.

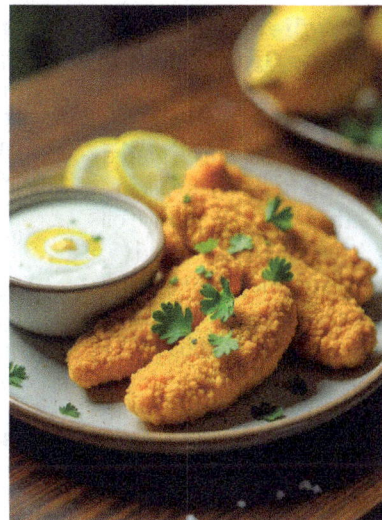

Nutritional Information (Per Serving):
- **Calories:** 260
- **Protein:** 30g
- **Carbohydrates:** 7g
- **Fats:** 13g
- **Fiber:** 2g
- **Cholesterol:** 70mg
- **Sodium:** 470mg
- **Potassium:** 500mg

BASIL & SPINACH PESTO CHICKEN

Yield: 4 servings • Prep Time: 10 minutes • Cook Time: 20–25 minutes • Total Time: 30–35 minutes

Ingredients:
For the Chicken:
> **4** boneless, skinless chicken breasts (about 1 lb or 450g)
> **1 tbsp** olive oil
> **1 tsp** sea salt (or to taste)
> **½ tsp** ground black pepper (to taste)
> **1 tsp** garlic powder (optional, for extra flavor)

For the Pesto:
> **2 cups** fresh basil leaves (packed)
> **1 cup** fresh spinach leaves (packed)
> **2 tbsp** olive oil (extra virgin)
> **1/4 cup** pine nuts (or walnuts for a more affordable alternative)
> **2 cloves** garlic (minced, anti-inflammatory properties)
> **¼ cup** grated Parmesan cheese (optional, or use nutritional yeast for a dairy-free version)
> **1 tbsp** lemon juice (adds vitamin C and antioxidants)
> **¼ tsp** sea salt (or to taste)
> **¼ tsp** black pepper

Instructions:
1. **Prep the Chicken:** Preheat your oven to 375°F (190°C). Rub the chicken breasts with olive oil, and season with sea salt, black pepper, and garlic powder (if using). Heat a large oven-safe skillet over medium heat, and once hot, sear the chicken breasts for about 3–4 minutes on each side, until golden brown. Once seared, transfer the skillet to the preheated oven and bake the chicken for 15–20 minutes, or until the chicken is cooked through (internal temperature should reach 165°F or 74°C).
2. **Make the Pesto:** While the chicken is cooking, prepare the pesto. In a food processor or blender, combine the fresh basil, spinach, pine nuts, garlic, lemon juice, olive oil, Parmesan (if using), sea salt, and black pepper. Pulse until smooth, scraping down the sides as needed. Add more olive oil if necessary to reach your desired consistency.
3. **Assemble the Dish:** Once the chicken is done baking, remove it from the oven and let it rest for a few minutes. Spoon the pesto over the chicken breasts, spreading it evenly across each piece.
4. **Serve:** Serve the chicken on a plate with a side of roasted vegetables, quinoa, or a simple green salad for a complete, anti-inflammatory meal.

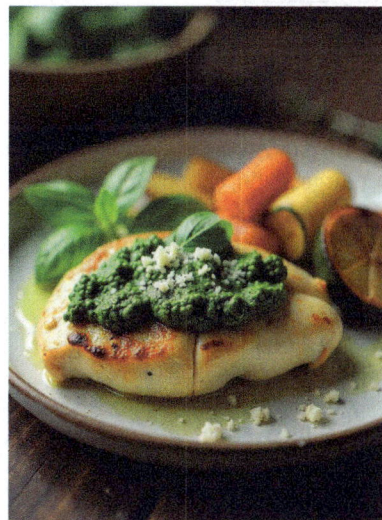

Nutritional Information (Per Serving):
- **Calories:** 350
- **Protein:** 35g
- **Carbohydrates:** 5g
- **Fats:** 22g
- **Fiber:** 2g
- **Cholesterol:** 70mg
- **Sodium:** 400mg
- **Potassium:** 600mg

GINGER-LEMON BAKED DRUMSTICKS

Yield: 4 servings • Prep Time: 15 minutes (plus 30 minutes to marinate) • Cook Time: 35-40 minutes • Total Time: 50-55 minutes

Ingredients:
For the Ginger-Lemon Marinade:
> **8** chicken drumsticks
> **2 tbsp** fresh ginger, grated
> **2 tbsp** fresh lemon juice
> **3 tbsp** extra virgin olive oil
> **3 garlic cloves**, minced
> **1 tbsp** honey (optional, for a touch of sweetness, choose raw honey for added benefits)
> **1 tbsp** apple cider vinegar
> **1 tsp** turmeric powder
> **1 tsp** ground cumin
> **1 tsp** smoked paprika (adds flavor, rich in antioxidants)
> Salt and freshly ground black pepper, to taste

Instructions:
1. **Prepare the Marinade:** In a medium bowl, whisk together the grated ginger, lemon juice, olive oil, garlic, honey (if using), apple cider vinegar, turmeric, cumin, smoked paprika, salt, and pepper.
2. **Marinate the Drumsticks:** Place the chicken drumsticks in a resealable plastic bag or shallow dish. Pour the marinade over the chicken, ensuring that each drumstick is evenly coated. Seal the bag or cover the dish and refrigerate for at least 30 minutes (up to 2 hours) to allow the flavors to infuse the chicken.
3. **Preheat the Oven:** Preheat your oven to 400°F (200°C). Line a baking sheet with parchment paper or lightly grease it with olive oil.
4. **Bake the Drumsticks:** Arrange the marinated drumsticks on the prepared baking sheet in a single layer. Bake for 35-40 minutes, flipping the drumsticks halfway through the cooking time to ensure even cooking. The drumsticks are done when the internal temperature reaches 165°F (74°C) and the juices run clear.
5. **Serve:** Once cooked, remove the drumsticks from the oven and let them rest for 5 minutes before serving. This helps retain the juiciness of the chicken.

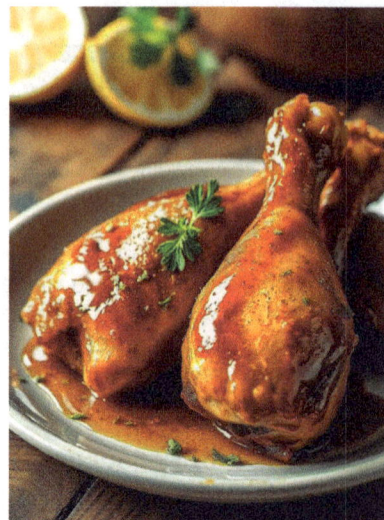

Nutritional Information (Per Serving, 2 drumsticks):
- **Calories:** 310
- **Protein:** 30g
- **Carbohydrates:** 9g
- **Fats:** 19g
- **Fiber:** 2g
- **Cholesterol:** 90mg
- **Sodium:** 350mg
- **Potassium:** 440mg

HEARTIER POULTRY DISHES

CHICKEN & SWEET POTATO CURRY WITH COCONUT

Yield: 4 servings • Prep Time: 15 minutes • Cook Time: 30 minutes • Total Time: 45 minutes

Ingredients:
For the Curry:
> **1 lb** (450g) boneless, skinless chicken breasts or thighs, cut into bite-sized pieces
> **2 tbsp** olive oil or coconut oil
> **1 large** onion, chopped
> **3 cloves** garlic, minced
> **1-inch** piece fresh ginger, grated
> **1 tbsp** ground turmeric
> **1 tsp** ground cumin
> **1 tsp** ground coriander
> **1/2 tsp** ground cinnamon
> **1/4 tsp** cayenne pepper
> **2 medium** sweet potatoes, peeled and diced into 1-inch cubes
> **1 can** (14 oz) full-fat coconut milk
> **1 cup** low-sodium chicken broth (or vegetable broth)
> Salt and freshly ground black pepper, to taste
For Garnish (Optional):
> Fresh cilantro, chopped
> Lime wedges
> A dollop of plain Greek yogurt or dairy-free yogurt (optional, for extra creaminess)

Instructions:
1. **Prepare the Ingredients:** Dice sweet potatoes into 1-inch cubes. Chop the chicken, onion, mince the garlic, and grate the ginger.
2. **Cook the Chicken:** Heat 1 tbsp oil in a large pot over medium heat. Add the chicken pieces and season with salt and pepper. Sauté for about 5-7 minutes until the chicken is browned and cooked through. Remove the chicken from the pot and set it aside.
3. **Sauté the Aromatics:** In the same pot, add the remaining 1 tbsp of oil. Add the chopped onion and sauté for 3-4 minutes until soft. Add garlic and ginger, cooking for 1-2 minutes while stirring.
4. **Add the Spices:** Add the turmeric, cumin, coriander, cinnamon, and cayenne pepper (if using) to the pot. Stir well to coat the onions and garlic in the spices. Cook for 1-2 minutes until fragrant.
5. **Add the Sweet Potatoes and Liquids:** Add the diced sweet potatoes to the pot, stirring to combine them with the spices. Pour in the coconut milk and chicken broth, and stir. Bring the mixture to a simmer.
6. **Simmer the Curry:** Reduce the heat to medium-low and cover the pot. Let it simmer for 15-20 minutes, or until the sweet potatoes are tender and the curry has thickened slightly.
7. **Finish the Dish:** Add the cooked chicken back into the pot and stir to combine. Simmer for an additional 5 minutes to ensure the chicken is heated through and the flavors meld together.
8. **Serve:** Ladle into bowls, garnish with cilantro and lime, and add yogurt if desired. Pair with brown rice, quinoa, or enjoy on its own.

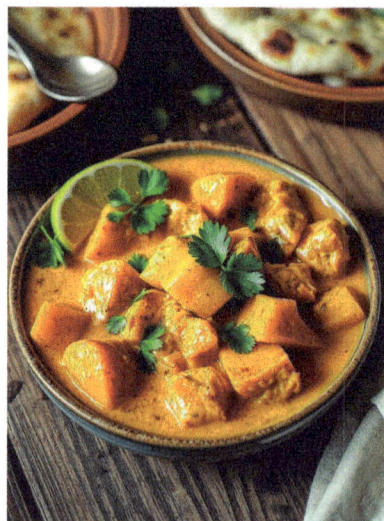

Nutritional Information (Per Serving):
- **Calories:** 370
- **Protein:** 32g
- **Carbohydrates:** 28g
- **Fats:** 18g
- **Fiber:** 6g
- **Cholesterol:** 70mg
- **Sodium:** 400mg
- **Potassium:** 950mg

TURKEY & SWEET POTATO CHILI

Yield: 6 servings • Prep Time: 15 minutes • Cook Time: 45 minutes • Total Time: 1 hour

Ingredients:
For the Chili:
> **1 lb** (450g) ground turkey breast
> **2 tbsp** olive oil
> **1 large** onion, diced
> **2 cloves** garlic, minced
> **1 medium** sweet potato, peeled and diced
> **1 can** (14.5 oz) diced tomatoes
> **1 can** (15 oz) kidney beans, drained and rinsed
> **1 can** (15 oz) black beans, drained and rinsed
> **1 cup** low-sodium chicken broth
> **1 tbsp** ground cumin
> **1 tsp** ground turmeric
> **1 tsp** smoked paprika
> **1/2 tsp** ground cinnamon
> **1/2 tsp** cayenne pepper (optional, for a spicy kick)
> Salt and pepper to taste

Optional Toppings:
> Fresh cilantro
> Sliced avocado
> Greek yogurt
> Shredded cheddar cheese

Instructions:
1. **Cook the Turkey:** Heat 1 tablespoon of olive oil in a large pot or Dutch oven over medium heat. Add the ground turkey and cook for 5-7 minutes, breaking it up with a spoon until browned. Remove any excess fat.
2. **Sauté the Vegetables:** In the same pot, add the remaining tablespoon of olive oil. Add the diced onion and garlic, sautéing for 3-4 minutes until softened and fragrant.
3. **Add the Sweet Potatoes and Spices:** Add the diced sweet potato to the pot and cook for 3-4 minutes, stirring occasionally. Sprinkle in the cumin, turmeric, smoked paprika, cinnamon, and cayenne pepper (if using). Stir to combine, allowing the spices to coat the vegetables and turkey.
4. **Simmer the Chili:** Add the diced tomatoes, kidney beans, black beans, and chicken broth to the pot. Stir everything together. Bring to a simmer, then reduce the heat to low. Cover and simmer for 30-35 minutes, stirring occasionally, until the sweet potatoes are tender and the chili has thickened.
5. **Season and Serve:** Taste and adjust the seasoning with salt and pepper, if needed. Serve the chili hot, and add any desired toppings such as fresh cilantro, avocado, Greek yogurt, or shredded cheese.

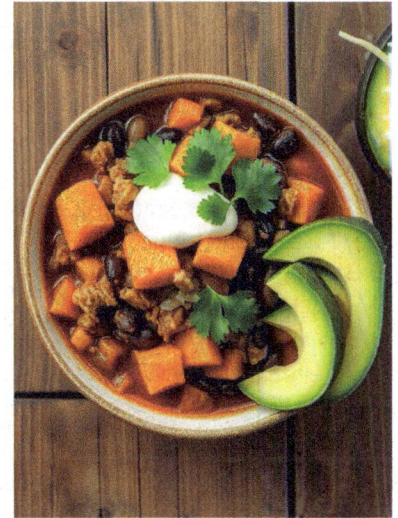

Nutritional Information (Per Serving):
- **Calories:** 350
- **Protein:** 28g
- **Carbohydrates:** 42g
- **Fats:** 11g
- **Fiber:** 9g
- **Cholesterol:** 80mg
- **Sodium:** 450mg
- **Potassium:** 900mg

BRAISED CHICKEN THIGHS WITH GINGER & CARROTS

Yield: 4 servings • Prep Time: 15 minutes • Cook Time: 1 hour • Total Time: 1 hour 15 minutes

Ingredients:
For the Braise:
> **4** turkey legs
> **2 tbsp** olive oil
> **1 medium** onion, chopped
> **4 cloves** garlic, minced
> **2 tbsp** fresh ginger, grated
> **1 1/2 tsp** ground turmeric
> **1 tsp** ground cumin
> **1/2 tsp** ground coriander
> **1/4 tsp** ground cinnamon
> **1 1/2 cups** low-sodium chicken or vegetable broth
> **1 tbsp** apple cider vinegar
> Salt and pepper to taste

Optional Ingredients for Garnish or Extra Flavor:
> Fresh cilantro, chopped
> A squeeze of fresh lemon juice
> **1/4 cup** sliced almonds

Instructions:
1. **Brown the Chicken Thighs:** Heat 1 tablespoon of olive oil in a large skillet or Dutch oven over medium-high heat. Season the chicken thighs with a pinch of salt and pepper. Add the chicken thighs, skin-side down, and brown for 4-5 minutes on each side until golden brown. Remove the chicken from the skillet and set aside.
2. **Sauté the Aromatics:** In the same skillet, add the remaining tablespoon of olive oil. Add the chopped onion and sauté for 3-4 minutes, or until softened. Add the minced garlic and sliced ginger, and cook for another 1-2 minutes until fragrant.
3. **Add the Carrots and Spices:** Add the sliced carrots, ground turmeric, cumin, black pepper, and cinnamon to the skillet, stirring to combine. Cook for 2-3 minutes, allowing the spices to toast and the carrots to soften slightly.
4. **Add the Liquid:** Pour in the chicken broth and apple cider vinegar, stirring to combine. Bring the mixture to a simmer.
5. **Braise the Chicken:** Return the browned chicken thighs to the skillet, skin-side up. Cover the skillet with a lid and reduce the heat to low. Let the chicken braise for 40-50 minutes, or until the chicken is tender and the carrots are fully cooked. Occasionally check to ensure the broth doesn't evaporate too much, adding a bit more chicken broth if necessary.
6. **Final Touches and Serve:** Once the chicken is tender, remove the lid and let the dish simmer for an additional 5-10 minutes to thicken the sauce. Taste and adjust seasoning with more salt or pepper as needed.
7. **Toppings:** For added freshness and a burst of flavor, top the dish with chopped fresh cilantro and a drizzle of plain Greek yogurt (if desired).

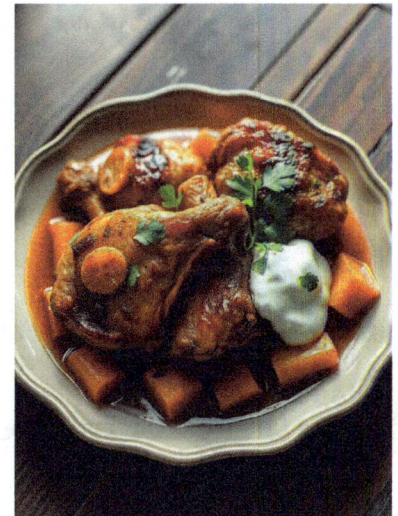

Nutritional Information (Per Serving):
- **Calories:** 375
- **Protein:** 30g
- **Carbohydrates:** 18g
- **Fats:** 22g
- **Fiber:** 4g
- **Cholesterol:** 85mg
- **Sodium:** 450mg
- **Potassium:** 800mg

TURMERIC & CUMIN BRAISED TURKEY LEGS

Yield: 4 servings • Prep Time: 15 minutes • Cook Time: 1 hour 30 minutes • Total Time: 1 hour 45 minutes

Ingredients:
For the Braise:
> 4 turkey legs
> 2 tbsp olive oil
> 1 medium onion, chopped
> 4 cloves garlic, minced
> 2 tbsp fresh ginger, grated
> 1 1/2 tsp ground turmeric
> 1 tsp ground cumin
> 1/2 tsp ground coriander
> 1/4 tsp ground cinnamon
> 1 1/2 cups low-sodium chicken or vegetable broth
> 1 tbsp apple cider vinegar
> Salt and pepper to taste

Optional Ingredients for Garnish or Extra Flavor:
> Fresh cilantro, chopped
> A squeeze of fresh lemon juice
> 1/4 cup sliced almonds

Instructions:
1. **Prepare the Turkey Legs:** Pat the turkey legs dry with paper towels and season generously with salt, pepper, turmeric, cumin, coriander, and cinnamon. Massage the spices into the turkey for even coating. 1 tbsp olive oil in a large skillet or Dutch oven over medium-high heat. Add turkey legs and brown on all sides, about 6–8 minutes. Remove and set aside.
2. **Sauté the Aromatics:** In the same pan, add the remaining 1 tablespoon of olive oil. Add the chopped onion and sauté for 3-4 minutes, until softened. Add the minced garlic and grated ginger, cooking for another 1-2 minutes until fragrant.
3. **Add the Liquid:** Pour in the chicken or vegetable broth and apple cider vinegar, stirring to combine. Scrape any browned bits from the bottom of the pan to incorporate into the liquid for more flavor.
4. **Braised Cooking:** Return the browned turkey legs to the pan, nestling them in the aromatics and broth. Bring the broth to a simmer, then reduce the heat to low. Cover the pan with a lid and braise the turkey legs for 1 hour to 1 hour 30 minutes, or until the turkey is tender and easily falls off the bone.
5. **Finish the Dish:** Once the turkey is fully cooked, remove the turkey legs from the pan and set them aside. If desired, reduce the sauce by simmering uncovered for 10-15 minutes to thicken. Taste the sauce and adjust the seasoning with additional salt or pepper if needed.
6. **Serve:** Serve the turkey legs over quinoa, brown rice, or roasted vegetables. Garnish with fresh cilantro, a squeeze of lemon juice, and optional sliced almonds for crunch.

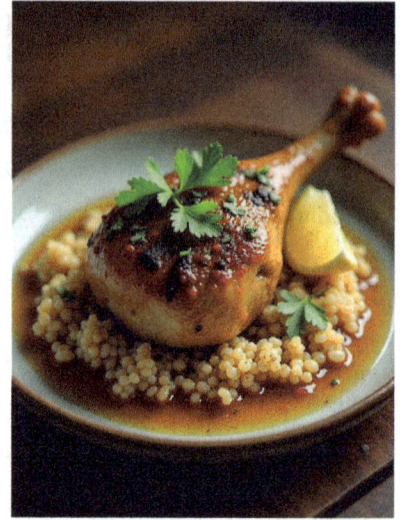

Nutritional Information (Per Serving):
- **Calories:** 320
- **Protein:** 40g
- **Carbohydrates:** 15g
- **Fats:** 15g
- **Fiber:** 3g
- **Cholesterol:** 135mg
- **Sodium:** 450mg
- **Potassium:** 560mg

COCONUT-CURRY TURKEY MEATBALLS

Yield: 4 servings • Prep Time: 15 minutes • Cook Time: 25 minutes • Total Time: 40 minutes

Ingredients:
For the Meatballs:
> 1 lb ground turkey breast
> 1/4 cup almond flour
> 1/4 cup chopped fresh cilantro
> 1 large egg
> 2 cloves garlic, minced
> 1/2 tsp ground turmeric
> 1/2 tsp ground cumin
> 1/4 tsp ground coriander
> Salt and pepper to taste
> 1 tbsp olive oil

For the Coconut-Curry Sauce:
> 1 can (14 oz) full-fat coconut milk
> 1 tbsp red curry paste
> 1 tsp ground turmeric
> 1 tsp ground ginger
> 1 tbsp lime juice
> 1 tbsp coconut oil
> 1/2 cup low-sodium chicken broth
> 1 tbsp honey
> Salt and pepper to taste

Optional Garnish:
> Chopped fresh cilantro
> Lime wedges
> A handful of toasted coconut flakes

Instructions:
1. **Prepare the Meatballs:** Preheat oven to 375°F (190°C) and line a baking sheet. Mix turkey, almond flour, cilantro, egg, garlic, spices, salt, and pepper. Shape into 16–18 meatballs. Place on the sheet, drizzle with olive oil, and bake for 20–25 minutes until golden and cooked through.
2. **Prepare the Coconut-Curry Sauce:** While the meatballs are baking, heat 1 tablespoon of coconut oil in a medium saucepan over medium heat. Add the red curry paste, ground turmeric, ground ginger, and a pinch of salt. Stir for 1-2 minutes until fragrant, allowing the spices to bloom. Pour in the coconut milk, chicken broth, lime juice, and honey (if using). Stir well to combine. Bring the sauce to a simmer, then reduce the heat to low. Let it simmer for 5-7 minutes, allowing the sauce to thicken slightly. Taste and adjust the seasoning with salt and pepper if needed.
3. **Combine and Serve:** Add baked meatballs to the sauce and simmer for 3–5 minutes. Serve with quinoa, cauliflower rice, or veggies.
4. **Optional Garnish:** Top with cilantro, toasted coconut, and lime juice as desired.

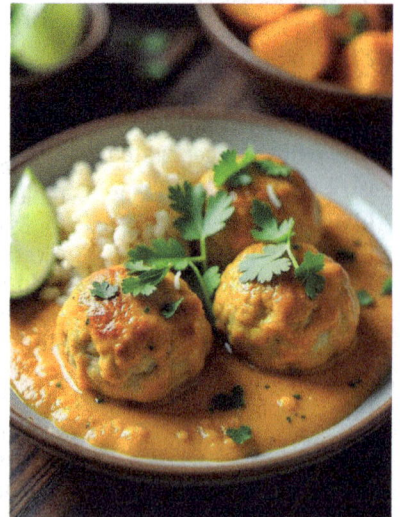

Nutritional Information (Per Serving):
- **Calories:** 375
- **Protein:** 28g
- **Carbohydrates:** 12g
- **Fats:** 24g
- **Fiber:** 4g
- **Cholesterol:** 120mg
- **Sodium:** 340mg
- **Potassium:** 680mg

ROASTED HERB CHICKEN WITH ROOT VEGETABLES

Yield: 4 servings • Prep Time: 15 minutes • Cook Time: 45 minutes • Total Time: 1 hour

Ingredients:
For the Chicken:
> **4** bone-in, skin-on chicken thighs (or breasts, if preferred) – 1 1/2 to 2 lbs
> **2 tbsp** olive oil
> **1 tbsp** fresh rosemary, finely chopped
> **1 tbsp** fresh thyme, finely chopped
> **1 tsp** ground turmeric
> **1 tsp** garlic powder
> **1/2 tsp** paprika
> **1/2 tsp** black pepper
> Salt to taste

For the Root Vegetables:
> **3 medium** carrots, peeled and cut into 1-inch pieces
> **2 medium** parsnips, peeled and cut into 1-inch pieces
> **2 medium** sweet potatoes, peeled and cut into 1-inch cubes
> **1 tbsp** olive oil
> **1/2 tsp** ground turmeric
> **1/2 tsp** ground cumin
> **1/2 tsp** ground cinnamon
> Salt and black pepper to taste

Optional Garnish:
> Chopped fresh parsley
> Lemon wedges

Instructions:
1. **Prepare the Chicken:** Preheat oven to 400°F (200°C). Mix olive oil, rosemary, thyme, turmeric, garlic powder, paprika, pepper, and salt into a paste. Pat chicken dry, rub with herb mixture, and marinate for 10 minutes.
2. **Prepare the Vegetables:** Toss carrots, parsnips, and sweet potatoes with olive oil, turmeric, cumin, cinnamon, salt, and pepper. Spread evenly on a baking sheet.
3. **Roast the Chicken and Vegetables:** Place the seasoned chicken thighs on top of the vegetables, skin side up. This will allow the chicken to release juices that flavor the vegetables. Roast in the preheated oven for 35-45 minutes, or until the chicken reaches an internal temperature of 165°F (75°C) and the vegetables are tender. You may want to check the vegetables and chicken at the 30-minute mark and stir the vegetables to ensure they cook evenly. If the chicken skin is not as crispy as desired, broil for the last 2-3 minutes of cooking to achieve a golden, crispy finish.
4. **Serve:** Let chicken rest for a few minutes. Plate with roasted vegetables and garnish with parsley and lemon juice if desired.

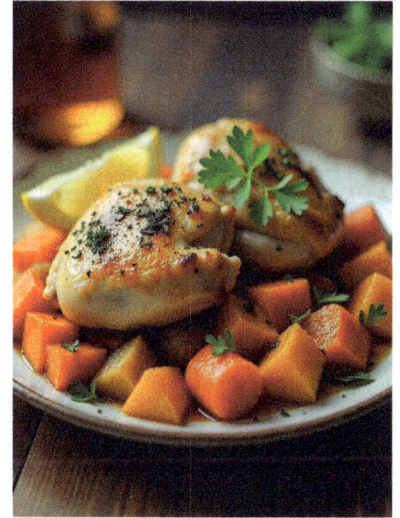

Nutritional Information (Per Serving):
- **Calories:** 420
- **Protein:** 34g
- **Carbohydrates:** 40g
- **Fats:** 18g
- **Fiber:** 8g
- **Cholesterol:** 120mg
- **Sodium:** 400mg
- **Potassium:** 1,100mg

ORANGE & GINGER GLAZED DUCK BREAST

Yield: 2 servings • Prep Time: 10 minutes • Cook Time: 25-30 minutes • Total Time: 35-40 minutes

Ingredients:
For the Duck Breast:
> **2** boneless, skin-on duck breasts (about 6 oz each)
> **1 tbsp** olive oil
> Salt and pepper to taste

For the Orange & Ginger Glaze:
> **1/2 cup** fresh orange juice
> **1 tbsp** fresh ginger, grated
> **1 tbsp** honey
> **1 tsp** ground turmeric
> **1 tbsp** apple cider vinegar
> **1/2 tsp** chili flakes

Optional Garnish:
> Fresh orange slices
> Fresh cilantro or parsley

Instructions:
1. **Prepare the Duck Breasts:** Pat the duck breasts dry with a paper towel to ensure crispy skin when cooked. Season both sides of the duck breasts with salt and pepper. Heat olive oil in a heavy skillet (preferably cast iron) over medium-high heat. Once the oil is hot, add the duck breasts, skin side down. Cook the duck breasts for about 6-8 minutes on the skin side until the skin is golden and crispy. Flip the duck breasts and reduce the heat to medium. Continue cooking for another 5-7 minutes (for medium-rare), or longer if you prefer them well-done. Once cooked, remove from the skillet and let rest for 5 minutes before slicing.
2. **Make the Orange & Ginger Glaze:** Simmer orange juice, ginger, honey, turmeric, vinegar, and chili flakes in a saucepan for 5–7 minutes until thickened.
3. **Serve:** Slice duck, drizzle with glaze, and garnish with orange slices or herbs. Serve with roasted vegetables or greens.

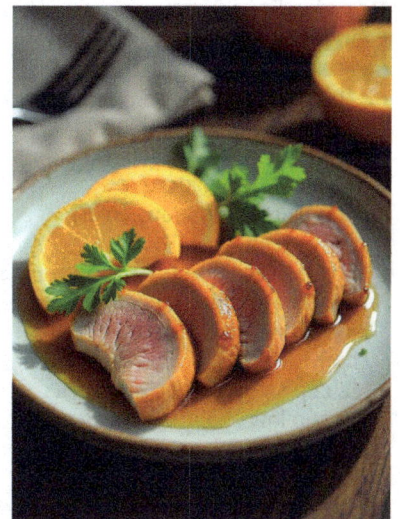

Nutritional Information (Per Serving):
- **Calories:** 350
- **Protein:** 27g
- **Carbohydrates:** 20g
- **Fats:** 24g
- **Fiber:** 3g
- **Cholesterol:** 75mg
- **Sodium:** 220mg
- **Potassium:** 460mg

7. MEAT RECIPES
LEAN MEATS

LEMON-ROSEMARY GRILLED LAMB CHOPS

Yield: 4 servings • Preparation Time: 10 minutes • Marinating Time: 30 minutes to 2 hours • Cooking Time: 10-12 minutes • Total Time: 40 minutes to 2 hours 12 minutes

Ingredients:
For the Lamb Chops:
> **4** lamb chops (about 6 oz each)
> **1 tbsp** olive oil
> Salt and pepper to taste

For the Marinade:
> **2 tbsp** fresh lemon juice
> **1 tbsp** lemon zest
> **2 garlic cloves**, minced
> **1 tbsp** fresh rosemary, finely chopped
> **1 tsp** dried oregano
> **1 tbsp** honey
> **1 tsp** ground turmeric
> **1/2 tsp** ground black pepper
> **1 tbsp** apple cider vinegar

Instructions:
1. **Prepare the Marinade:** In a small bowl, whisk together the lemon juice, lemon zest, minced garlic, rosemary, oregano, honey, turmeric, black pepper, and apple cider vinegar. Season the lamb chops with salt and pepper, then place them in a shallow dish or resealable plastic bag. Pour the marinade over the lamb chops, ensuring they are well coated. Seal the dish or bag and refrigerate for 30 minutes to 2 hours.
2. **Preheat the Grill:** Preheat the grill or grill pan over medium-high heat (about 400°F/200°C). Lightly oil the grates or pan with olive oil.
3. **Grill the Lamb Chops:** Remove the lamb chops from the marinade and let them sit at room temperature for a few minutes. Grill the lamb chops for about 4-5 minutes per side, depending on your preferred doneness (medium-rare to medium). Use a meat thermometer to ensure the internal temperature reaches 125°F for rare or 145°F for medium. Turn the chops halfway through grilling to ensure even cooking.
4. **Rest and Serve:** Let the lamb chops rest for 5 minutes before serving to allow the juices to redistribute. Serve with anti-inflammatory side dishes such as roasted vegetables or a fresh green salad.

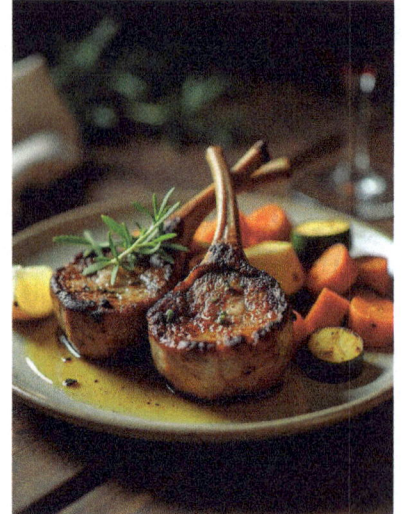

Nutritional Information (Per Serving):
- **Calories:** 350
- **Protein:** 30g
- **Carbohydrates:** 8g
- **Fats:** 24g
- **Fiber:** 2g
- **Cholesterol:** 80mg
- **Sodium:** 250mg
- **Potassium:** 450mg

BEEF & VEGGIE STIR-FRY WITH GINGER

Yield: 4 servings • Preparation Time: 10 minutes • Cooking Time: 10-12 minutes • Total Time: 20 minutes

Ingredients:
For the Stir-Fry:
> **1 lb** (450g) grass-fed beef, thinly sliced
> **2 tbsp** olive oil
> **1 medium** red onion, thinly sliced
> **2 cloves** garlic, minced
> **1 cup** bell peppers (any color), thinly sliced
> **1 cup** broccoli florets (or cauliflower if preferred)
> **1 medium** carrot, julienned or thinly sliced
> **1/2 cup** snap peas or snow peas
> **1/4 cup** low-sodium soy sauce or coconut aminos
> **1 tbsp** apple cider vinegar
> **1-2 tbsp** fresh ginger, grated
> **1 tbsp** sesame oil
> **1/2 tsp** ground turmeric
> Salt and pepper to taste

Optional Garnishes:
> Fresh cilantro or parsley for garnish
> Sesame seeds for added texture
> Sliced green onions for a fresh flavor kick

Instructions:
1. **Prepare the Ingredients:** Slice beef thinly, chop vegetables (onion, bell peppers, broccoli, carrot, snap peas), grate ginger, and mince garlic.
2. **Cook the Beef:** Heat 1 tablespoon of olive oil (or avocado oil) in a large skillet or wok over medium-high heat. Add the beef in batches (to avoid overcrowding) and cook for 3-4 minutes per side until browned and just cooked through. Remove the beef from the skillet and set aside.
3. **Sauté the Vegetables:** In the same skillet, add the remaining tablespoon of oil. Add the onion and garlic and sauté for 1-2 minutes until fragrant. Add the bell peppers, broccoli, carrot, and snap peas to the pan. Stir-fry for 4-5 minutes, allowing the vegetables to soften slightly but still retain their crunch. If needed, add a splash of water to create steam and help soften the veggies.
4. **Add Flavor:** Once the vegetables are cooked, add the grated ginger, turmeric, soy sauce (or coconut aminos), and apple cider vinegar (if using). Stir everything together and cook for another 1-2 minutes, ensuring the vegetables are evenly coated in the sauce and spices.
5. **Combine and Serve:** Add beef back, stir, and heat through. Adjust salt and pepper as needed.
6. **Serve:** Garnish with cilantro, sesame seeds, or green onions. Enjoy warm!

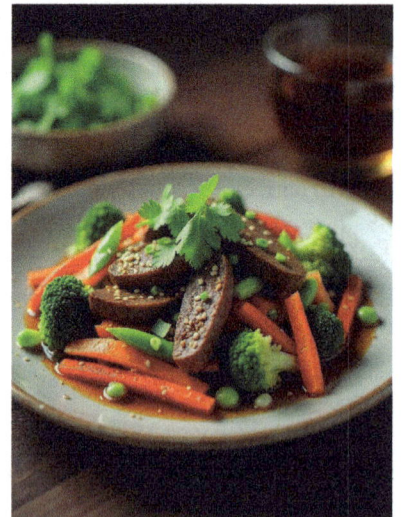

Nutritional Information (Per Serving):
- **Calories:** 290
- **Protein:** 30g
- **Carbohydrates:** 15g
- **Fats:** 14g
- **Fiber:** 4g
- **Cholesterol:** 60mg
- **Sodium:** 450mg (with low-sodium soy sauce)
- **Potassium:** 600mg

PORK TENDERLOIN WITH APPLE-MUSTARD GLAZE

Yield: 4 servings • Preparation Time: 10 minutes • Cooking Time: 25-30 minutes • Total Time: 35-40 minutes

Ingredients:
For the Pork Tenderloin:
> **1 lb** (450g) pork tenderloin
> **2 tbsp** olive oil
> Salt and pepper to taste
> **1 tsp** dried thyme
> **1 tsp** garlic powder

For the Apple-Mustard Glaze:
> **1/2 cup** unsweetened apple cider (or apple juice)
> **2 tbsp** Dijon mustard
> **1 tbsp** apple cider vinegar
> **1 tbsp** honey
> **1/2 tsp** ground turmeric
> **1/4 tsp** ground cinnamon
> **1 tbsp** fresh lemon juice
> **1/2 tsp** sea salt or to taste
> Fresh parsley for garnish (optional)

Instructions:
1. **Prepare the Pork Tenderloin:** Preheat the oven to 400°F (200°C). Pat the pork tenderloin dry with paper towels and season it evenly with salt, pepper, garlic powder, and dried thyme. Heat 1 tablespoon of olive oil in a large oven-safe skillet over medium-high heat. Once the oil is hot, sear the pork tenderloin for 2-3 minutes on each side until browned and caramelized.
2. **Make the Apple-Mustard Glaze:** In a small saucepan, combine the apple cider (or apple juice), Dijon mustard, apple cider vinegar, honey (if using), turmeric, cinnamon, and lemon juice. Stir well to combine. Bring the mixture to a simmer over medium heat. Reduce the heat and continue simmering for 5-7 minutes, stirring occasionally, until the glaze thickens slightly. Taste the glaze and adjust the seasoning with salt, pepper, or honey if needed.
3. **Roast the Pork:** Drizzle 2 tbsp glaze over seared pork, then roast in the oven for 15–20 minutes, basting occasionally, until internal temp reaches 145°F (63°C). While the pork is roasting, occasionally baste with more of the apple-mustard glaze for added flavor.
4. **Finish the Dish:** Rest pork for 5–10 minutes, slice, and drizzle with remaining glaze. Garnish with parsley if desired.

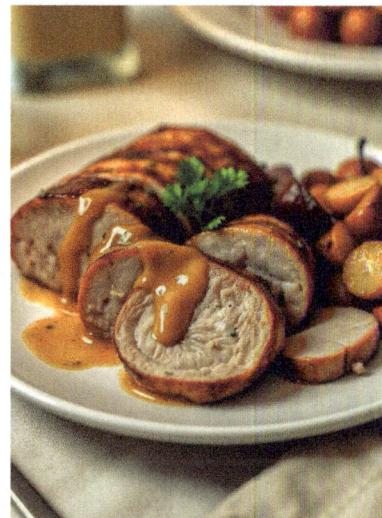

Nutritional Information (Per Serving):
- **Calories:** 285
- **Protein:** 32g
- **Carbohydrates:** 15g
- **Fats:** 12g
- **Fiber:** 2g
- **Cholesterol:** 80mg
- **Sodium:** 430mg
- **Potassium:** 650mg

LEAN BEEF SKEWERS WITH BELL PEPPERS

Yield: 4 servings • Preparation Time: 15 minutes (plus 30 minutes for marinating) • Cooking Time: 10-12 minutes • Total Time: 40-45 minutes

Ingredients:
For the Skewers:
> **1 lb** lean beef (sirloin, flank, or tenderloin), cut into 1-inch cubes
> **2 large** bell peppers (any color), cut into 1-inch pieces
> **1** red onion, cut into 1-inch pieces
> **2 tbsp** olive oil
> **1 tbsp** balsamic vinegar
> **1 tbsp** fresh lemon juice
> Salt and pepper, to taste

For the Marinade:
> **2 tbsp** olive oil
> **2 garlic cloves**, minced
> **1 tsp** ground turmeric
> **1/2 tsp** ground cumin
> **1/2 tsp** paprika
> **1/4 tsp** ground black pepper
> **1 tsp** dried oregano
> **1/2 tsp** red pepper flakes

Optional Toppings:
> Fresh parsley or cilantro, chopped
> A squeeze of fresh lime juice

Instructions:
1. **Prepare the Marinade:** Mix olive oil, garlic, turmeric, cumin, paprika, oregano, black pepper, and red pepper flakes.
2. **Marinate the Beef:** Place the beef cubes in a shallow dish or resealable plastic bag. Pour the marinade over the beef and toss to coat evenly. Seal the dish or bag and refrigerate for at least 30 minutes, allowing the flavors to meld and the beef to absorb the anti-inflammatory properties of the marinade.
3. **Prepare the Skewers:** Cut bell peppers and onions into 1-inch pieces. Thread beef, peppers, and onions onto skewers.
4. **Cook the Skewers:** Preheat a grill or grill pan to medium-high heat. Brush the grill with a little olive oil to prevent sticking. Place the skewers on the grill and cook for about 10-12 minutes, turning occasionally, until the beef reaches your desired level of doneness (about 145°F for medium-rare). If using a grill pan, cook in batches to avoid overcrowding.
5. **Serve:** Rest skewers for a few minutes, then garnish with parsley or cilantro and a squeeze of lime juice.

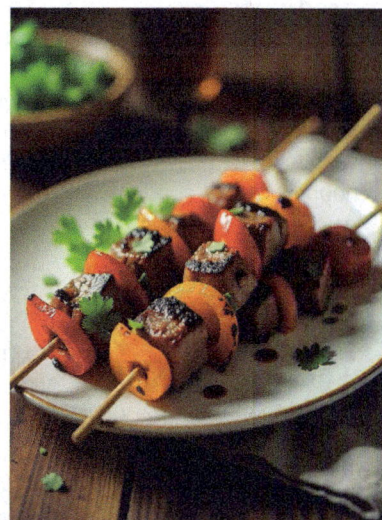

Nutritional Information (Per Serving):
- **Calories:** 280
- **Protein:** 30g
- **Carbohydrates:** 15g
- **Fats:** 14g
- **Fiber:** 4g
- **Cholesterol:** 70mg
- **Sodium:** 320mg
- **Potassium:** 500mg

GRILLED PORK CHOPS WITH FRESH HERBS

Yield: 4 servings • Prep Time: 15 minutes (plus 30 minutes to marinate) • Cooking Time: 10-12 minutes • Total Time: 55 minutes

Ingredients:
For the Herb Marinade:
› **4** bone-in pork chops (6 oz each)
› **2 tbsp** extra virgin olive oil
› **1 tbsp** fresh rosemary, finely chopped
› **1 tbsp** fresh thyme, finely chopped
› **2 garlic cloves**, minced
› **1 tsp** ground turmeric
› **1/2 tsp** ground black pepper
› **1 tbsp** apple cider vinegar
› **1 tsp** Dijon mustard
› **1/2 tsp** sea salt (or to taste)

Optional Toppings (for added taste and nutrition):
› Freshly chopped parsley
› Lemon wedges
› A drizzle of honey

Instructions:
1. **Prepare the Marinade:** In a small bowl, whisk together the olive oil, rosemary, thyme, minced garlic, turmeric, black pepper, apple cider vinegar, Dijon mustard, and sea salt. Whisk until smooth and well combined.
2. **Marinate the Pork Chops:** Place the pork chops in a shallow dish or resealable plastic bag. Pour the marinade over the pork chops, making sure they are evenly coated. Cover the dish or seal the bag, then refrigerate for at least 30 minutes to allow the flavors to meld. For a stronger flavor, marinate for up to 2 hours.
3. **Grill the Pork Chops:** Preheat a grill or grill pan to medium-high heat. If using a grill pan, lightly brush it with olive oil to prevent sticking. Remove the pork chops from the marinade, letting any excess marinade drip off. Place the pork chops on the grill and cook for 5-6 minutes per side, or until they reach an internal temperature of 145°F for medium doneness. Remove the pork chops from the grill and allow them to rest for a few minutes to retain their juices.
4. **Serve:** Plate the pork chops and optionally top with fresh parsley, a squeeze of lemon juice, and a light drizzle of honey. Serve with a side salad or grilled vegetables for added fiber and nutrients.

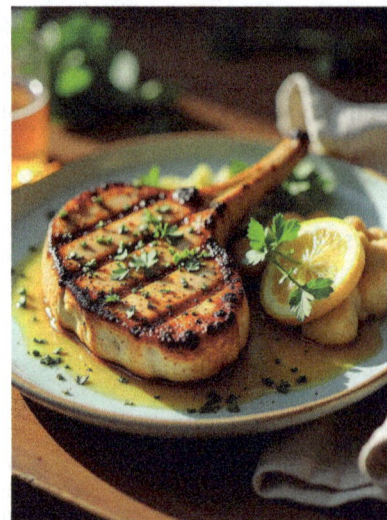

Nutritional Information (Per Serving):
- **Calories**: 310
- **Protein**: 28g
- **Carbohydrates**: 3g
- **Fats**: 20g
- **Fiber**: 1g
- **Cholesterol**: 80mg
- **Sodium**: 450mg
- **Potassium**: 530mg

ROASTED VENISON WITH GARLIC & THYME

Yield: 4 servings • Prep Time: 10 minutes (plus 30 minutes for marinating) • Cooking Time: 20-25 minutes • Total Time: 55 min

Ingredients:
For the Marinade:
› **1 lb** venison loin or tenderloin, trimmed of excess fat
› **2 tbsp** extra virgin olive oil
› **1 tbsp** fresh thyme, finely chopped
› **3 garlic cloves**, minced
› **1 tsp** apple cider vinegar
› **1/2 tsp** ground black pepper
› **1/2 tsp** sea salt

For Roasting:
› **1 tbsp** extra virgin olive oil
› **1/2 tsp** ground rosemary

Optional Toppings:
› Fresh thyme sprigs
› A squeeze of fresh lemon juice

Instructions:
1. **Prepare the Marinade:** In a small bowl, mix together 2 tbsp olive oil, fresh thyme, minced garlic, apple cider vinegar, black pepper, and sea salt. Whisk until the marinade is smooth and well combined.
2. **Marinate the Venison:** Place the venison in a shallow dish or large resealable bag. Pour the marinade over the venison, ensuring it is evenly coated. Cover the dish or seal the bag and refrigerate for at least 30 minutes. Marinating for up to 2 hours will further infuse the flavors.
3. **Roast the Venison:** Preheat your oven to 400°F (200°C). In a large oven-safe skillet, heat 1 tbsp olive oil over medium-high heat. Remove the venison from the marinade, letting any excess drip off. Sear the venison for 2-3 minutes on each side until browned. Sprinkle with ground rosemary if using, then transfer the skillet to the preheated oven. Roast for 15-20 minutes or until the internal temperature reaches 130°F (54°C) for medium-rare, or adjust to your preferred level of doneness.
4. **Rest and Serve:** Remove the venison from the oven and let it rest in the skillet for 5 minutes to retain its juices. Slice the venison and plate, garnishing with fresh thyme and a light squeeze of lemon juice for added flavor and anti-inflammatory benefits.

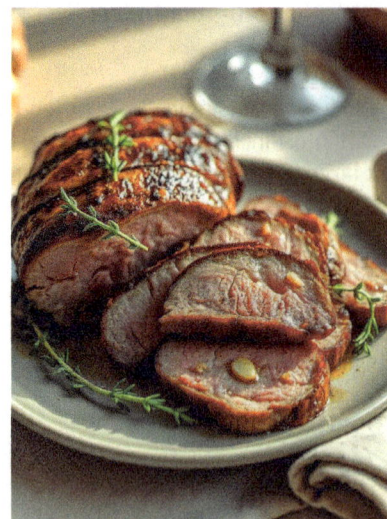

Nutritional Information (Per Serving):
- **Calories**: 230
- **Protein**: 30g
- **Carbohydrates**: 1g
- **Fats**: 11g
- **Fiber**: 0g
- **Cholesterol**: 85mg
- **Sodium**: 350mg
- **Potassium**: 600mg

COMFORT MEAT DISHES

BRAISED BEEF WITH CARROTS AND CELERY

Yield: 4 servings • Preparation Time: 15 minutes • Cooking Time: 2.5 - 3 hours (including passive simmering time) • Total Time: 3 hours, 15 minutes

Ingredients:
For the Braise:
> **1 lb** lean beef chuck, trimmed of excess fat and cut into 1.5-inch cubes
> **1 tbsp** extra virgin olive oil
> **1 medium** onion, chopped
> **3 garlic cloves**, minced
> **2 large** carrots, peeled and cut into 1-inch rounds
> **2 stalks** celery, cut into 1-inch pieces
> **1 tsp** ground turmeric
> **1/2 tsp** ground black pepper
> **1/2 tsp** ground cumin
> **1/2 tsp** dried thyme
> **1/2 tsp** dried rosemary
> **1/4 tsp** sea salt (or to taste)
> **1 cup** low-sodium beef broth
> **1 cup** water

Optional Ingredients:
> **1/2 cup** mushrooms, sliced

Instructions:
1. **Prepare the Ingredients:** Cut the beef chuck into 1.5-inch cubes. Chop the onions, garlic, carrots, and celery.
2. **Sear the Beef:** In a large heavy-bottomed pot or Dutch oven, heat the olive oil over medium-high heat. Add the beef cubes in a single layer, searing each side for 2-3 minutes until browned. Remove beef and set aside.
3. **Sauté Aromatics:** Lower the heat to medium and add the chopped onion to the pot. Sauté for 3-4 minutes until translucent. Add the minced garlic and cook for another 1 minute until fragrant.
4. **Add Vegetables and Spices:** Stir in the carrots, celery, turmeric, black pepper, cumin, thyme, rosemary, and sea salt. Cook for 2-3 minutes to let the vegetables and spices combine.
5. **Deglaze and Add Liquids:** Add the beef broth to the pot, scraping up any brown bits stuck to the bottom (this adds flavor). Add the beef cubes back into the pot and pour in enough water to cover the ingredients by about 1 inch.
6. **Simmer the Braise:** Bring the pot to a gentle boil, then reduce the heat to low, covering the pot with a lid. Allow it to simmer for 2.5 - 3 hours, or until the beef is tender and the flavors have melded. Stir occasionally and add a bit more water if it becomes too thick.
7. **Finish and Serve:** Taste and adjust seasonings if necessary. Garnish with fresh parsley, if using. Serve warm, optionally with a side of whole grains or leafy greens.

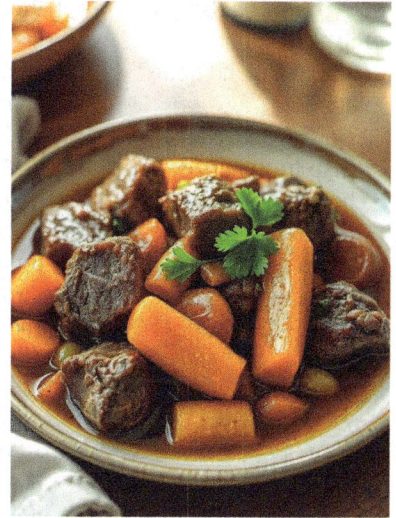

Nutritional Information (Per Serving):
- **Calories**: 300
- **Fiber**: 3g
- **Protein**: 27g
- **Cholesterol**: 60mg
- **Carbohydrates**: 10g
- **Sodium**: 370mg
- **Fats**: 17g
- **Potassium**: 690mg

MEATLOAF WITH ALMOND FLOUR

Yield: 4 servings • Preparation Time: 15 minutes • Cooking Time: 1 hour • Total Time: 1 hour, 15 minutes

Ingredients:
> **1 lb** lean ground turkey
> **1/2 cup** almond flour
> **1 small** onion, finely diced
> **1 medium** carrot, grated
> **2 cloves** garlic, minced
> **1 tbsp** fresh parsley, chopped
> **1 tbsp** fresh thyme, chopped
> **1 tsp** turmeric powder
> **1/2 tsp** smoked paprika
> **1/2 tsp** sea salt (or to taste)
> **1/4 tsp** black pepper

For the Topping:
> **2 tbsp** tomato paste
> **1 tsp** apple cider vinegar
> **1 tsp** honey

Instructions:
1. **Preheat the Oven**: Preheat your oven to 350°F (175°C). Grease a loaf pan lightly or line it with parchment paper for easy removal.
2. **Prepare the Meatloaf Mixture**: In a large mixing bowl, combine the ground turkey, almond flour, onion, grated carrot, garlic, parsley, thyme, turmeric, smoked paprika, salt, and black pepper. Mix well until all ingredients are evenly incorporated.
3. **Shape the Meatloaf**: Transfer the mixture to the prepared loaf pan and press it evenly to form a loaf shape.
4. **Prepare the Topping**: In a small bowl, mix together the tomato paste, apple cider vinegar, and honey (if using). Spread this mixture evenly over the top of the meatloaf for a tangy, antioxidant-rich glaze.
5. **Bake**: Place the meatloaf in the preheated oven and bake for 50-60 minutes, or until the internal temperature reaches 165°F (74°C). Let it rest for a few minutes before slicing.
6. **Serve**: Slice the meatloaf and serve warm. Optionally, garnish with additional fresh parsley for extra flavor and antioxidants.

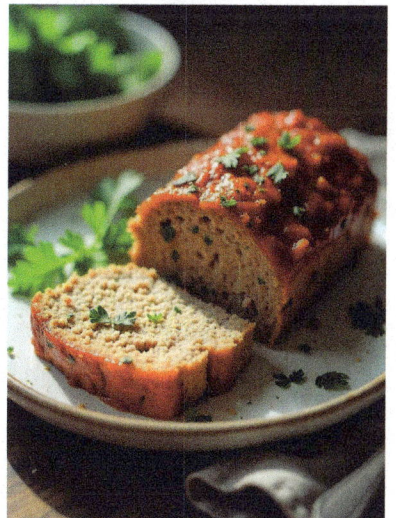

Nutritional Information (Per Serving):
- **Calories**: 270
- **Fiber**: 4g
- **Protein**: 28g
- **Cholesterol**: 70mg
- **Carbohydrates**: 10g
- **Sodium**: 410mg
- **Fats**: 14g
- **Potassium**: 600mg

HONEY & TURMERIC PORK MEATBALLS

Yield: 4 servings (approx. 4-5 meatballs per serving) • Preparation Time: 15 minutes • Cooking Time: 20 minutes • Total Time: 35 minutes

Ingredients:
For the Meatballs:
> **1 lb** ground pork
> **1/4 cup** almond flour
> **1 egg**
> **2 cloves** garlic, minced
> **1 tbsp** fresh parsley, finely chopped
> **1 tsp** ground turmeric
> **1/2 tsp** ground black pepper
> **1/2 tsp** sea salt (or to taste)
> **1/4 tsp** cayenne pepper

For the Glaze:
> **1 tbsp** honey
> **1 tbsp** apple cider vinegar
> **1/2 tsp** ground turmeric
> **1/4 tsp** ground black pepper

Instructions:
1. **Prepare the Meatballs**: Preheat the oven to 375°F (190°C). In a large bowl, combine the ground pork, almond flour, egg, garlic, parsley, turmeric, black pepper, sea salt, and cayenne pepper (if using). Use your hands to mix everything together until evenly combined. Roll the mixture into meatballs, about 1-1.5 inches in diameter, and place them on a baking sheet lined with parchment paper or lightly greased with olive oil.
2. **Bake the Meatballs**: Place the meatballs in the preheated oven and bake for 15-20 minutes, or until they are cooked through and reach an internal temperature of 160°F (71°C). The outside should be golden and crispy.
3. **Prepare the Glaze**: While the meatballs are baking, whisk together the honey, apple cider vinegar, turmeric, and black pepper in a small bowl until smooth. Set aside.
4. **Glaze the Meatballs**: Once the meatballs are done baking, remove them from the oven. Drizzle the prepared glaze over the meatballs, or toss them gently to coat each meatball evenly with the glaze.
5. **Serve**: Serve the meatballs hot with a side of vegetables or over a bed of quinoa for a complete anti-inflammatory meal. Optionally, garnish with fresh parsley or cilantro.

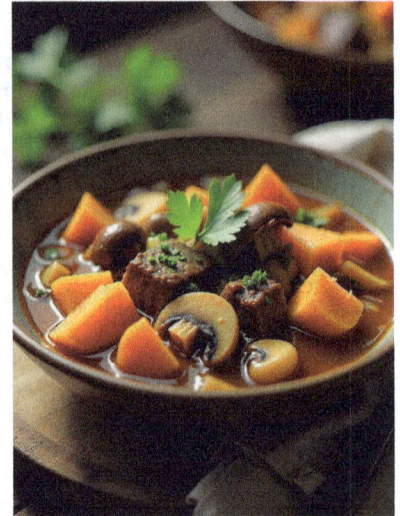

Nutritional Information (Per Serving - 4-5 Meatballs):
- **Calories**: 240
- **Fiber**: 2g
- **Protein**: 18g
- **Cholesterol**: 75mg
- **Carbohydrates**: 8g
- **Sodium**: 500mg
- **Fats**: 16g
- **Potassium**: 380mg

HEARTY BEEF STEW WITH MUSHROOMS

Yield: 4 servings • Preparation Time: 20 minutes • Cooking Time: 2 hours (includes passive simmering time) • Total Time: 2 hours 20 minutes

Ingredients:
For the Stew:
> **1 lb** lean beef stew meat, cut into 1-inch cubes
> **1 tbsp** olive oil
> **1 medium** onion, diced
> **3 cloves** garlic, minced
> **2 medium** carrots, sliced
> **2 celery** stalks, sliced
> **1 cup** mushrooms, sliced
> **1 medium** sweet potato, diced
> **1 cup** low-sodium beef broth
> **1 cup** water
> **1 tbsp** tomato paste
> **1 tsp** dried thyme
> **1 tsp** dried rosemary
> **1/2 tsp** ground turmeric
> **1/2 tsp** black pepper
> **1/2 tsp** sea salt (or to taste)

Optional Additions:
> **1/4 cup** fresh parsley, chopped
> A squeeze of fresh lemon juice

Instructions:
1. **Prepare the Beef**: In a large pot or Dutch oven, heat the olive oil over medium-high heat. Add the beef cubes and sear on all sides until browned (about 5-7 minutes). This browning process locks in the flavors. Remove the beef from the pot and set aside.
2. **Sauté the Vegetables**: In the same pot, cook onions and garlic for 3 minutes. Add carrots, celery, and mushrooms, cooking for 5 more minutes.
3. **Add the Remaining Ingredients**: Return the browned beef to the pot. Add the diced sweet potato, beef broth, water, and tomato paste. Stir well to combine. Sprinkle in the thyme, rosemary, turmeric, black pepper, and sea salt, mixing thoroughly to incorporate the spices.
4. **Simmer the Stew**: Bring to a boil, reduce heat, cover, and simmer for 1.5–2 hours until beef is tender.
5. **Serve**: Ladle into bowls and garnish with parsley and lemon juice.

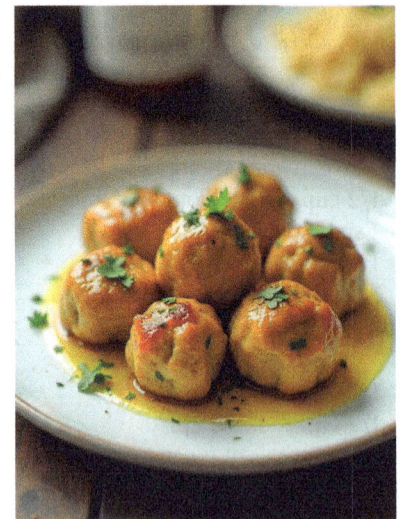

Nutritional Information (Per Serving):
- **Calories**: 320
- **Fiber**: 5g
- **Protein**: 28g
- **Cholesterol**: 70mg
- **Carbohydrates**: 24g
- **Sodium**: 320mg
- **Fats**: 12g
- **Potassium**: 800mg

GINGER & GARLIC MARINATED LAMB STEW

Yield: 4 servings • Preparation Time: 15 minutes • Marinating Time: 30 minutes (or up to 2 hours for enhanced flavor) • Cooking Time: 1 hour 30 minutes (includes passive simmering) • Total Time: 2 hours 15 minutes

Ingredients:
For the Marinade:
> **1 lb** lamb stew meat, cut into 1-inch cubes
> **1 tbsp** fresh ginger, grated
> **3 cloves** garlic, minced
> **1 tbsp** olive oil
> **1 tbsp** apple cider vinegar
> **1/2 tsp** sea salt (or to taste)
> **1/2 tsp** ground black pepper

For the Stew:
> **1 tbsp** olive oil
> **1 medium** onion, diced
> **2 medium** carrots, sliced
> **1 cup** mushrooms, sliced
> **1 medium** zucchini, diced
> **2 cups** low-sodium beef or vegetable broth
> **1 cup** water
> **1 tsp** turmeric powder
> **1/2 tsp** cumin powder
> **1/2 tsp** ground coriander
> **1/2 tsp** ground cinnamon
> **1** bay leaf
> **Optional: 1/4 cup** chopped fresh parsley

Instructions:
1. **Marinate the Lamb:** Combine lamb with grated ginger, garlic, olive oil, apple cider vinegar, salt, and pepper. Marinate for 30 minutes to 2 hours.
2. **Sauté the Aromatics**: In a large pot or Dutch oven, heat 1 tbsp of olive oil over medium heat. Add the diced onion and cook until it becomes translucent, about 3-4 minutes. Add the carrots, mushrooms, and zucchini, and cook for another 5 minutes, stirring occasionally.
3. **Add the Lamb and Spices**: Remove the lamb from the marinade and add it to the pot, browning it on all sides for about 5 minutes. Add the turmeric, cumin, coriander, and cinnamon, stirring to coat the meat and vegetables in the spices.
4. **Simmer the Stew**: Add broth, water, and bay leaf. Bring to a boil, then reduce heat and simmer for 1-1.5 hours until lamb is tender.
5. **Serve**: Remove bay leaf, garnish with parsley, and serve.

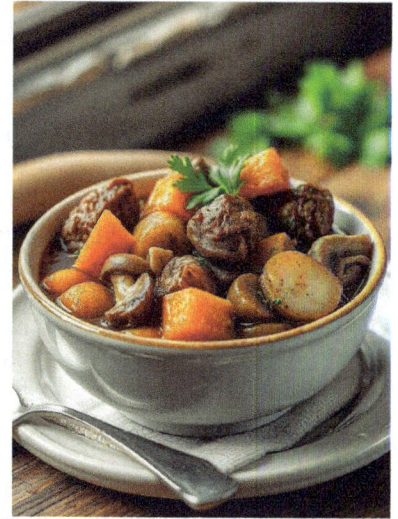

Nutritional Information (Per Serving):
- **Calories**: 330
- **Protein**: 27g
- **Carbohydrates**: 15g
- **Fats**: 18g
- **Fiber**: 5g
- **Cholesterol**: 70mg
- **Sodium**: 320mg
- **Potassium**: 800mg

SPICED BEEF & LENTIL CASSEROLE

Yield: 4 servings • Preparation Time: 15 minutes • Cooking Time: 45 minutes (includes simmering) • Total Time: 1 hour

Ingredients:
For the Casserole:
> **1 lb** lean grass-fed ground beef
> **1 tbsp** olive oil
> **1 medium** onion, diced
> **2 garlic cloves**, minced
> **1 large** carrot, diced
> **1 tsp** ground turmeric
> **1 tsp** ground cumin
> **1/2 tsp** ground cinnamon
> **1/2 tsp** ground black pepper
> **1 cup** green or brown lentils, rinsed
> **1 can** (14 oz) diced tomatoes, no salt added
> **2 cups** low-sodium beef or vegetable broth
> **1** bay leaf
> **1/2 tsp** sea salt (or to taste)
> **1/4 cup** fresh parsley, chopped

Optional Toppings:
> Fresh cilantro, chopped
> Sliced avocado
> Lemon wedges

Instructions:
1. **Sauté the Aromatics**: Heat the olive oil in a large pot or Dutch oven over medium heat. Add the onion and garlic, and sauté until softened, about 5 minutes. Add the diced carrot and cook for another 3-4 minutes.
2. **Add the Spices**: Stir in the ground turmeric, cumin, cinnamon, and black pepper, and cook for 1-2 minutes, allowing the spices to become fragrant.
3. **Brown the Beef**: Add the ground beef to the pot and cook until browned, breaking it up with a spoon as it cooks, about 5-7 minutes.
4. **Add Lentils, Tomatoes, and Broth**: Stir in the lentils, diced tomatoes, and broth. Add the bay leaf and sea salt, and bring the mixture to a simmer.
5. **Simmer the Casserole**: Reduce the heat to low, cover, and let the casserole simmer for about 30 minutes, or until the lentils are tender and the flavors have melded. Stir occasionally and add a little more broth or water if needed to keep the casserole moist.
6. **Serve**: Remove the bay leaf and stir in the chopped parsley. Serve the casserole warm, garnished with fresh cilantro, sliced avocado, or a squeeze of lemon juice for added flavor.

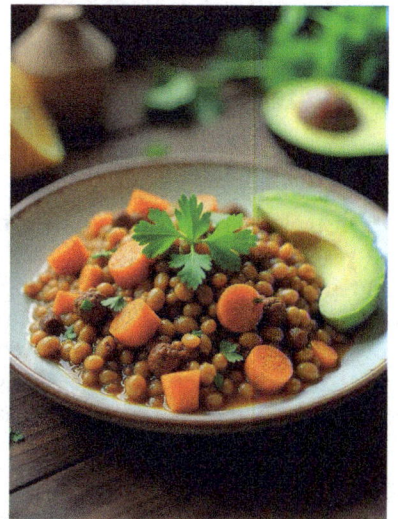

Nutritional Information (Per Serving):
- **Calories**: 420
- **Protein**: 30g
- **Carbohydrates**: 30g
- **Fats**: 16g
- **Fiber**: 9g
- **Cholesterol**: 70mg
- **Sodium**: 320mg
- **Potassium**: 850mg

8.VEGETABLE RECIPES
ROASTED & BAKED VEGETABLES

TURMERIC-ROASTED CAULIFLOWER WITH TAHINI DRIZZLE

Yield: 4 servings • Preparation Time: 10 minutes • Cooking Time: 25-30 minutes

Ingredients:
For the Roasted Cauliflower:
> **1 large** head of cauliflower (about 4 cups florets), cut into bite-sized pieces
> **2 tbsp** olive oil
> **1 ½ tsp** ground turmeric
> **1 tsp** ground cumin
> **1 tsp** paprika
> **½ tsp** garlic powder
> **½ tsp** black pepper
> Salt, to taste

For the Tahini Drizzle:
> **3 tbsp** tahini
> **1 tbsp** fresh lemon juice
> **1 tbsp** warm water
> **1 tsp** maple syrup or honey
> **1 small** garlic clove, minced
> Pinch of salt, to taste
> Fresh cilantro or parsley (for garnish)

Instructions:
1. **Preheat the Oven**: Preheat your oven to 400°F (200°C). Line a baking sheet with parchment paper for easy cleanup.
2. **Season the Cauliflower**: In a large bowl, toss the cauliflower florets with olive oil, turmeric, cumin, paprika, garlic powder (if using), black pepper, and salt. Ensure that the cauliflower is evenly coated with the spices and oil.
3. **Roast the Cauliflower**: Spread the seasoned cauliflower florets in a single layer on the prepared baking sheet. Roast in the preheated oven for 25-30 minutes, or until the cauliflower is tender and golden brown, flipping halfway through for even roasting.
4. **Mix the Drizzle**: In a small bowl, whisk together the tahini, lemon juice, warm water, maple syrup or honey (if using), garlic (if using), and a pinch of salt. Continue whisking until smooth. Adjust the consistency by adding more water if needed.
5. **Assemble the Dish**: Once the cauliflower is roasted, transfer it to a serving plate. Drizzle the tahini mixture over the top.
6. **Garnish**: Garnish with freshly chopped cilantro or parsley for an added burst of flavor and color.

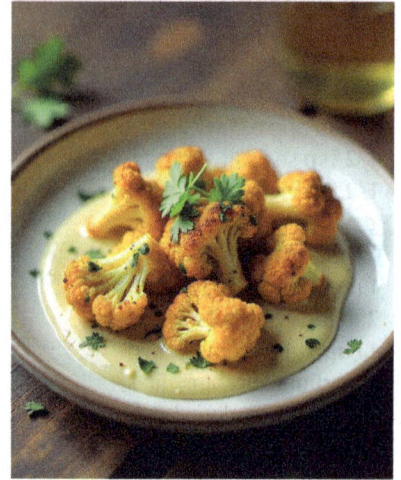

Nutritional Information (per serving):
- **Calories**: 190 kcal
- **Protein**: 4 g
- **Carbohydrates**: 14 g
- **Fats**: 14 g
- **Saturated Fat**: 2 g
- **Monounsaturated Fat**: 10 g
- **Fiber**: 5 g
- **Cholesterol**: 0 mg
- **Sodium**: 140 mg
- **Potassium**: 450 mg

SMOKY PAPRIKA SWEET POTATO WEDGES

Yield: 4 servings • Preparation Time: 10 minutes • Cooking Time: 30-35 minutes

Ingredients:
> **2 large** sweet potatoes, peeled and cut into wedges (about 4 cups)
> **2 tbsp** olive oil
> **1 ½ tsp** smoked paprika
> **1 tsp** ground turmeric
> **½ tsp** garlic powder
> **½ tsp** ground cumin
> **½ tsp** black pepper
> **½ tsp** sea salt (or to taste)
> **1 tbsp** fresh parsley, chopped (for garnish)

Instructions:
1. **Preheat the Oven**: Preheat your oven to 400°F (200°C). Line a baking sheet with parchment paper or lightly grease with olive oil to prevent sticking.
2. **Prepare the Sweet Potatoes**: Peel the sweet potatoes and cut them into wedges. Aim for uniform thickness so they cook evenly.
3. **Season the Wedges**: In a large bowl, toss the sweet potato wedges with olive oil, smoked paprika, turmeric, garlic powder (if using), cumin, black pepper, and salt. Ensure the wedges are evenly coated with the spices and oil mixture.
4. **Arrange and Roast**: Spread the seasoned sweet potato wedges in a single layer on the prepared baking sheet. Roast in the preheated oven for 30-35 minutes, flipping the wedges halfway through, until they are tender on the inside and crispy on the outside. The exact cooking time may vary depending on the size of the wedges, so check for doneness by piercing a wedge with a fork–it should go through easily.
5. **Garnish and Serve**: Once roasted, remove the sweet potato wedges from the oven and transfer them to a serving dish. Garnish with freshly chopped parsley for added color and flavor.

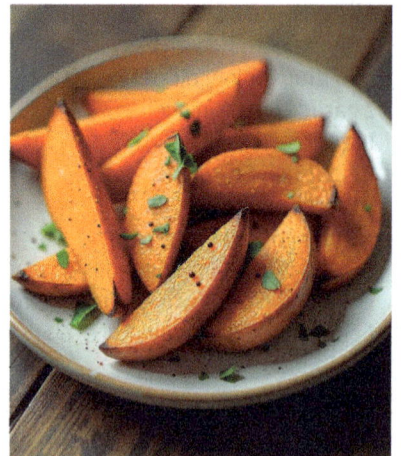

Nutritional Information (per serving):
- **Calories**: 180 kcal
- **Protein**: 3 g
- **Carbohydrates**: 36 g
- **Fats**: 5 g
- **Saturated Fat**: 0.5 g
- **Monounsaturated Fat**: 3.5 g
- **Fiber**: 6 g
- **Cholesterol**: 0 mg
- **Sodium**: 250 mg
- **Potassium**: 620 mg

LEMON & HERB ROASTED BRUSSELS SPROUTS

Yield: 4 servings • Preparation Time: 10 minutes • Cooking Time: 25-30 minutes

Ingredients:
For the Brussels Sprouts:
> **1 lb** (450g) Brussels sprouts, trimmed and halved
> **2 tbsp** extra virgin olive oil
> **2 cloves** garlic, minced
> Zest of 1 lemon
> **2 tbsp** fresh lemon juice
> **1 tsp** dried oregano
> **1 tsp** dried thyme ½ tsp sea salt
> **½ tsp** freshly ground black pepper

Optional Toppings:
> Fresh parsley, chopped
> Grated Parmesan or nutritional yeast
> Toasted pine nuts
> Balsamic glaze

Instructions:
1. **Preheat the Oven:** Preheat your oven to 400°F (200°C). Line a baking sheet with parchment paper or lightly grease it with olive oil.
2. **Prepare the Brussels Sprouts:** Trim the tough ends of the Brussels sprouts and remove any yellow or damaged outer leaves. Slice the Brussels sprouts in half for even cooking.
3. **Season the Brussels Sprouts:** In a large mixing bowl, toss the halved Brussels sprouts with olive oil, minced garlic, lemon zest, lemon juice, oregano, thyme, sea salt, and black pepper. Toss everything together until the Brussels sprouts are evenly coated with the seasoning mixture.
4. **Roast the Brussels Sprouts:** Spread sprouts on baking sheet and roast for 25-30 minutes, flipping halfway, until golden and crispy.
5. **Serve:** Garnish with parsley, Parmesan (or nutritional yeast), toasted pine nuts, and balsamic glaze if desired.

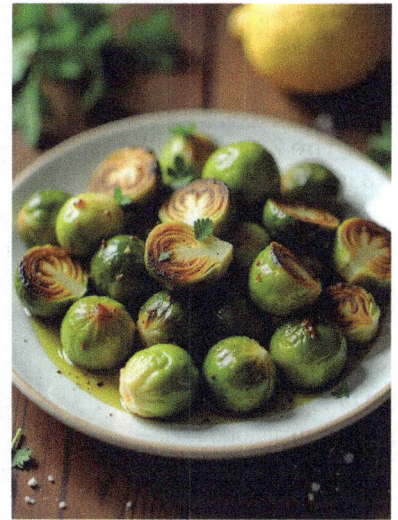

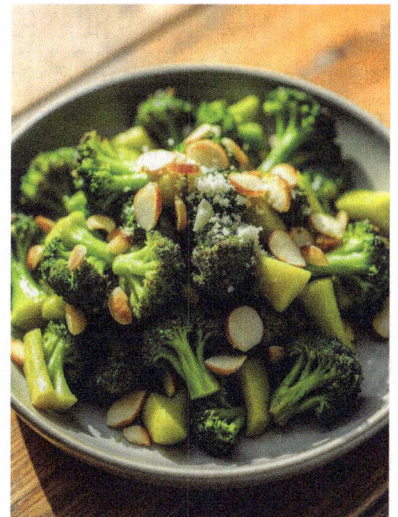

Nutritional Information (per serving):
- **Calories**: 160 kcal
- **Protein**: 4 g
- **Carbohydrates**: 15 g
- **Fiber**: 6 g
- **Sugars**: 3 g
- **Fats**: 11 g
- **Saturated Fat**: 1.5 g
- **Monounsaturated Fat**: 7 g
- **Cholesterol**: 0 mg
- **Sodium**: 250 mg
- **Potassium**: 400 mg
- **Vitamin C**: 80% of the daily value
- **Fiber**: 6 g (helps with digestion and gut health)

GARLIC & OLIVE OIL ROASTED BROCCOLI

Yield: 4 servings • Preparation Time: 10 minutes • Cooking Time: 20-25 minutes

Ingredients:
For the Roasted Broccoli:
> **1 lb** (450g) fresh broccoli, cut into florets
> **2 tbsp** extra virgin olive oil
> **3 cloves** garlic, minced
> **½ tsp** sea salt (or to taste)
> **¼ tsp** freshly ground black pepper
> **¼ tsp** red pepper flakes
> **1 tbsp** fresh lemon juice

Optional Toppings:
> Fresh lemon zest
> Grated Parmesan cheese (or nutritional yeast for a dairy-free option, adds a savory, nutty taste)
> Toasted almonds or pine nuts
> Fresh parsley or basil, chopped

Instructions:
1. **Preheat the Oven:** Heat oven to 400°F (200°C) and line a baking sheet with parchment paper.
2. **Prepare the Broccoli:** Trim the broccoli into small, even florets for consistent roasting. You can also peel and slice the stems to use them as well, as they are nutritious and tender when roasted.
3. **Season the Broccoli:** In a large mixing bowl, toss the broccoli florets with olive oil, minced garlic, sea salt, freshly ground black pepper, and red pepper flakes (if using). Make sure the broccoli is evenly coated with the oil and seasoning.
4. **Roast the Broccoli:** Spread sprouts on baking sheet and roast for 25-30 minutes, flipping halfway, until golden and crispy.
5. **Finish with Lemon:** Once roasted, remove the broccoli from the oven and squeeze fresh lemon juice over the top for a burst of flavor and antioxidants. For extra zest, you can also sprinkle some lemon zest.
6. **Serve:** Garnish with parsley, Parmesan (or nutritional yeast), toasted pine nuts, and balsamic glaze if desired.

Nutritional Information (per serving):
- **Calories**: 150 kcal
- **Protein**: 4 g
- **Carbohydrates**: 12 g
- **Fats**: 10 g
- **Saturated Fat**: 1.5 g
- **Monounsaturated Fat**: 8 g
- **Fiber**: 5 g
- **Cholesterol**: 0 mg
- **Sodium**: 200 mg
- **Potassium**: 600 mg

OVEN-BAKED ZUCCHINI FRIES WITH FRESH DILL

Yield: 4 servings • Preparation Time: 15 minutes • Cooking Time: 25-30 minutes

Ingredients:

For the Zucchini Fries:

> **3 medium** zucchinis, cut into 1/2-inch thick strips
> **2 tbsp** extra virgin olive oil
> **1/2 tsp** turmeric powder 1/4 tsp garlic powder
> **1/4 tsp** smoked paprika
> **1/4 tsp** ground black pepper
> **1/4 tsp** sea salt
> **1/4 cup** almond flour
> **1/4 cup** nutritional yeast

For the Fresh Dill Dip:

> **1/2 cup** Greek yogurt
> **1 tbsp** fresh dill, finely chopped
> **1 tsp** lemon juice
> **1/2 tsp** garlic powder
> Pinch of sea salt

Instructions:

1. **Preheat the Oven:** Heat oven to 425°F (220°C) and line a baking sheet with parchment paper.
2. **Prepare the Zucchini:** Cut off the ends and slice them into 1/2-inch thick strips, resembling fries. Pat them dry with a paper towel to remove any moisture, ensuring they crisp up in the oven.
3. **Season the Zucchini Fries:** Toss the zucchini strips with olive oil, turmeric, garlic powder, smoked paprika, black pepper, and sea salt. If you're using almond flour for extra crunch, toss the zucchini in it now. Optionally, sprinkle the zucchini with nutritional yeast for a cheesy flavor.
4. **Arrange on the Baking Sheet:** Place the seasoned zucchini strips in a single layer on the prepared baking sheet. Make sure they are not overcrowded, which will allow them to bake evenly and become crispy.
5. **Bake the Zucchini Fries:** Arrange zucchini in a single layer on the baking sheet. Bake for 25-30 minutes, flipping halfway through.
6. **Prepare the Fresh Dill Dip:** While the zucchini fries are baking, prepare the dip. In a small bowl, combine the Greek yogurt, fresh dill, lemon juice, garlic powder, and a pinch of sea salt. Mix well until smooth and creamy.
7. **Serve:** Serve the crispy zucchini fries with the fresh dill dip.

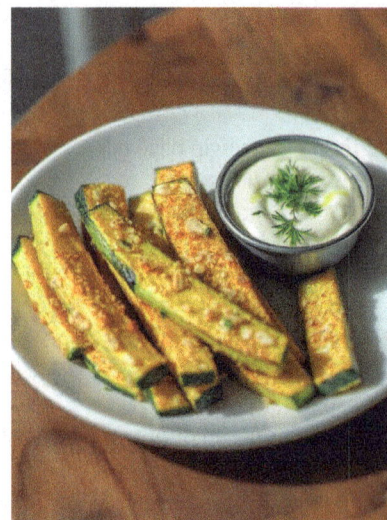

Nutritional Information (per serving):

- **Calories**: 140 kcal
- **Protein**: 6 g
- **Carbohydrates**: 12 g
- **Fats**: 10 g
- **Fiber**: 3 g
- **Cholesterol**: 5 mg
- **Sodium**: 220 mg
- **Potassium**: 400 mg

ROSEMARY & GARLIC ROASTED MUSHROOMS

Yield: 4 servings • Preparation Time: 10 minutes • Cooking Time: 25-30 minutes

Ingredients:

> **16 oz** (450g) cremini mushrooms or button mushrooms, cleaned and trimmed
> **2 tbsp** extra virgin olive oil
> **3 garlic cloves**, minced
> **1 tbsp** fresh rosemary, finely chopped
> **1/2 tsp** dried thyme
> **1/4 tsp** ground black pepper
> **1/4 tsp** sea salt
> **1 tsp** lemon juice

Optional Add-ins (for extra flavor and nutritional benefits):

> **1 tablespoon** balsamic vinegar
> **1 tablespoon** nutritional yeast

Instructions:

1. **Preheat the Oven**: Preheat your oven to 400°F (200°C). Line a baking sheet with parchment paper for easy cleanup.
2. **Prepare the Mushrooms**: Wipe the mushrooms clean with a damp cloth to remove any dirt, then trim the stems if needed. Cut larger mushrooms in half or quarters to ensure even cooking.
3. **Season the Mushrooms**: Toss mushrooms with olive oil, garlic, rosemary, thyme, black pepper, and sea salt.
4. **Arrange the Mushrooms**: Spread the seasoned mushrooms in a single layer on the prepared baking sheet. Make sure the mushrooms are evenly spaced to allow them to roast properly and become crispy on the edges.
5. **Roast the Mushrooms**: Spread mushrooms on the baking sheet. Roast for 25-30 minutes, stirring halfway through, until golden and tender.
6. **Finishing Touch**: Drizzle with lemon juice and, if desired, balsamic vinegar and nutritional yeast.
7. **Serve**: Serve hot as a side dish or on salads and bowls.

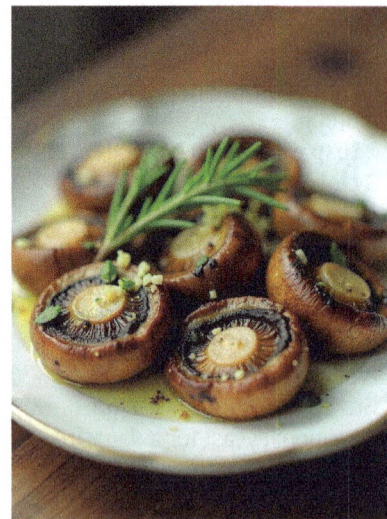

Nutritional Information (per serving):

- **Calories**: 120 kcal
- **Protein**: 2.5 g
- **Carbohydrates**: 10 g
- **Fats**: 9 g
- **Fiber**: 3 g
- **Cholesterol**: 0 mg
- **Sodium**: 220 mg
- **Potassium**: 500 mg

VEGETABLE SOUPS & STEWS

CREAMY CASHEW BROCCOLI SOUP WITH FRESH DILL

Yield: 4 servings • Preparation Time: 10 minutes • Cooking Time: 25–30 minutes

Ingredients:
For the Soup:
> **1 tbsp** extra virgin olive oil
> **1 medium** onion, diced
> **3 cloves** garlic, minced
> **4 cups** broccoli florets
> **3 cups** vegetable broth
> **1/2 cup** raw cashews, soaked for at least 2 hours
> **1 tsp** ground turmeric
> **1/2 tsp** ground black pepper
> **1/2 tsp** ground cumin
> **1/4 tsp** ground coriander
> **1/2 tsp** sea salt (to taste)
> **1/2 tsp** lemon zest
> **1 tbsp** fresh lemon juice

Optional Garnishes:
> Fresh dill, chopped
> A drizzle of olive oil or a dollop of dairy-free yogurt for extra creaminess
> Toasted sunflower seeds or pumpkin seeds for a crunchy topping

Instructions:
1. **Soak the Cashews:** Soak cashews in warm water for at least 2 hours. Drain before using.
2. **Prepare the Vegetables:** Heat the olive oil in a large pot over medium heat. Add the diced onion and sauté for 4-5 minutes, until softened and translucent. Add the minced garlic and sauté for another 30 seconds until fragrant.
3. **Cook the Broccoli:** Add the broccoli florets to the pot and stir for a minute. Pour in the vegetable broth and bring to a simmer. Cover the pot and cook for 10-15 minutes, or until the broccoli is tender.
4. **Blend the Soup:** Once the broccoli is tender, add the soaked and drained cashews to the pot. Stir in the turmeric, cumin, coriander, salt, lemon zest, and lemon juice. Use an immersion blender to blend the soup until smooth and creamy. If you don't have an immersion blender, carefully transfer the soup to a regular blender in batches and blend until smooth. Return the soup to the pot.
5. **Adjust Consistency:** If the soup is too thick, you can add a little more vegetable broth or water to reach your desired consistency. Stir well to combine.
6. **Taste and Adjust Seasonings:** Taste the soup and adjust the seasoning as needed, adding more salt, lemon juice, or turmeric if desired.
7. **Serve:** Garnish with fresh dill, olive oil, or toppings of choice.

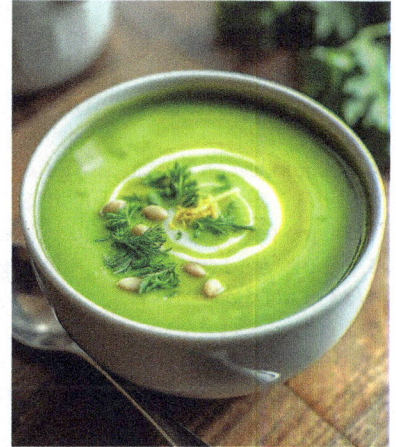

Nutritional Information (per serving): *(Please note: the values are approximate and based on the recipe as written, without optional toppings)*

- **Calories**: 290 kcal
- **Protein**: 8 g
- **Carbohydrates**: 21 g
- **Fats**: 22 g
- **Fiber**: 4 g
- **Cholesterol**: 0 mg
- **Sodium**: 500 mg (depending on vegetable broth and salt used)
- **Potassium**: 750 mg

TURMERIC VEGETABLE SOUP

Yield: 4 servings • Preparation Time: 15 minutes • Cooking Time: 30 minutes

Ingredients:
For the Soup:
> **1 Tbsp** olive oil
> **1 medium** onion, diced
> **3 cloves** garlic, minced
> **2 medium** carrots, peeled and diced
> **2 medium** zucchini, diced
> **1 cup** cauliflower florets
> **1 cup** broccoli florets
> **1 medium** potato, peeled and diced
> **1 tsp** ground turmeric
> **1/2 tsp** ground cumin
> **1/2 tsp** ground coriander
> **1/2 tsp** ground black pepper
> **1/2 tsp** sea salt (to taste)
> **1/4 tsp** cayenne pepper
> **4 cups** vegetable broth
> **1 cup** coconut milk
> **1 Tbsp** fresh lemon juice
> Fresh cilantro for garnish

Instructions:
1. **Prepare the Vegetables:** Peel, wash, and dice the carrots, zucchini, cauliflower, broccoli, and potato into bite-sized pieces. Set aside.
2. **Sauté Aromatics:** In a large pot, heat 1 Tbsp of olive oil over medium heat. Add the diced onion and cook for about 4-5 minutes, stirring occasionally, until the onion becomes soft and translucent. Add the minced garlic and cook for an additional 30 seconds, until fragrant.
3. **Add Vegetables and Spices:** Add carrots, zucchini, cauliflower, broccoli, and potato. Stir in turmeric, cumin, coriander, black pepper, salt, and cayenne pepper. Cook for 2-3 minutes.
4. **Add Broth and Simmer:** Pour in the vegetable broth and bring the mixture to a boil. Once boiling, reduce the heat to low and let the soup simmer for about 20-25 minutes, or until the vegetables are tender.
5. **Blend the Soup:** Once the vegetables are tender, use an immersion blender to blend the soup until smooth and creamy. Alternatively, you can carefully transfer the soup in batches to a regular blender, blend it, and return it to the pot.
6. **Add Coconut Milk and Lemon Juice:** Stir in 1 cup of coconut milk for a creamy texture and additional anti-inflammatory fat. Add the fresh lemon juice to brighten up the flavor and enhance detoxification.
7. **Taste and Adjust Seasoning:** Taste the soup and adjust the seasoning, adding more salt, pepper, or lemon juice as desired.
8. **Serve:** Ladle the soup into bowls, garnish with fresh cilantro, and enjoy!

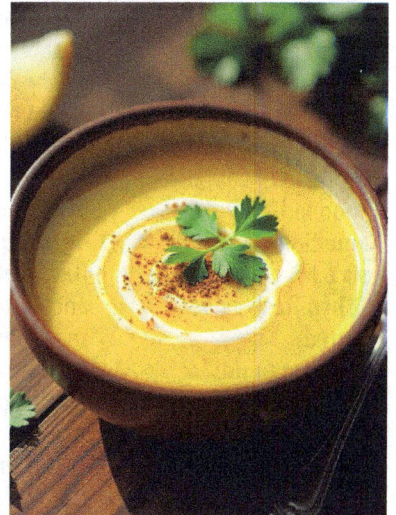

Nutritional Information (per serving):

- **Calories**: 210
- **Protein**: 4g
- **Carbohydrates**: 35g
- **Fats**: 10g
- **Saturated fat**: 7g
- **Fiber**: 6g
- **Cholesterol**: 0mg
- **Sodium**: 400mg
- **Potassium**: 800mg

ROASTED RED PEPPER AND TOMATO BASIL SOUP

Yield: 4 servings • Preparation Time: 15 minutes • Cooking Time: 40 minutes

Ingredients:
For the Soup:
> **1 Tbsp** olive oil
> **1 large** onion, chopped
> **3 cloves** garlic, minced
> **2** red bell peppers, roasted and peeled
> **4 medium** tomatoes, diced
> **1/2 tsp** ground turmeric
> **1/2 tsp** ground cumin
> **1/2 tsp** dried oregano
> **1/2 tsp** sea salt (to taste)
> **1/4 tsp** black pepper
> **4 cups** vegetable broth
> **1 cup** coconut milk
> **1 Tbsp** fresh lemon juice
> **1/4 cup** fresh basil leaves, chopped

Instructions:
1. **Roast the Red Peppers:** Preheat the oven to 400ºF (200ºC). Place the red bell peppers on a baking sheet and roast them for 20-25 minutes, turning occasionally, until the skins are charred. Once roasted, remove the peppers from the oven and let them cool. Peel off the skins, remove the seeds, and chop them into smaller pieces. Set aside.
2. **Sauté Aromatics:** In a large pot, heat olive oil over medium heat. Sauté onion for 4-5 minutes until soft. Add garlic and cook for 30 seconds.
3. **Add Vegetables and Spices:** Add the chopped roasted red peppers and diced tomatoes to the pot. Stir in the ground turmeric, cumin, oregano, salt, and black pepper. Cook for another 2-3 minutes, allowing the spices to release their flavors.
4. **Simmer:** Add vegetable broth, bring to a boil, then reduce heat and simmer for 20-25 minutes.
5. **Blend the Soup:** Use an immersion blender to blend the soup until smooth and creamy. Alternatively, transfer the soup to a regular blender in batches, blend until smooth, and return it to the pot.
6. **Add Coconut Milk and Lemon Juice:** Stir in 1 cup of coconut milk and 1 Tbsp fresh lemon juice for a creamy texture and a zesty kick. Let the soup simmer for an additional 5 minutes to combine the flavors.
7. **Add Fresh Basil:** Stir in fresh basil, adjust seasoning, and serve hot. Garnish with extra basil if desired. Enjoy!

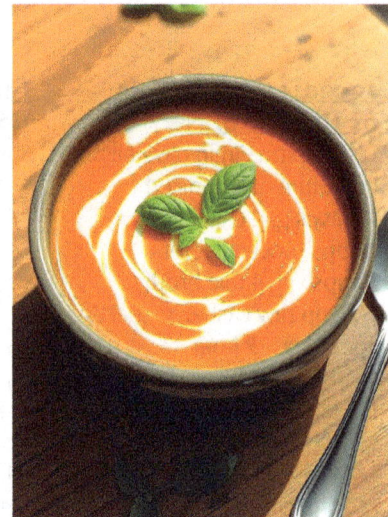

Nutritional Information (per serving):
- **Calories**: 210
- **Protein**: 4g
- **Carbohydrates**: 30g
- **Fats**: 12g
- **Saturated fat**: 6g
- **Fiber**: 6g
- **Cholesterol**: 0mg
- **Sodium**: 350mg
- **Potassium**: 750mg

CABBAGE & CELERY DETOX SOUP

Yield: 4 servings • Preparation Time: 15 minutes • Cooking Time: 30 minutes

Ingredients:
For the Soup:
> **1 Tbsp** olive oil
> **1 medium** onion, diced
> **2 cloves** garlic, minced
> **1 stalk** celery, chopped
> **1/2 head** of cabbage, chopped
> **2 medium** carrots, sliced
> **1 Tbsp** fresh ginger, grated
> **1/2 tsp** ground turmeric
> **1/2 tsp** ground cumin
> **1 (14.5 oz) can** diced tomatoes
> **4 cups** vegetable broth
> Salt and pepper, to taste

Instructions:
1. **Sauté Aromatics:** Heat olive oil in a large pot over medium heat. Add onion and cook for 3-4 minutes. Stir in garlic and ginger, cooking for 1-2 minutes until fragrant.
2. **Add Vegetables and Spices:** Add the chopped celery, carrots, and cabbage to the pot. Stir to combine with the aromatics, then add the ground turmeric, cumin, salt, and pepper. Cook for 2-3 minutes to allow the spices to release their flavors.
3. **Add Liquids:** Pour in the diced tomatoes with their juices and the vegetable broth. Bring to a boil, then reduce the heat to low and let the soup simmer, uncovered, for 20-25 minutes or until the vegetables are tender.
4. **Blend (Optional):** For a smooth soup, blend using an immersion blender or regular blender. For a chunkier soup, leave it as is.
5. **Taste and Adjust:** Taste the soup and adjust seasoning with salt and pepper if needed.
6. **Serve:** Ladle into bowls, garnish with fresh parsley or cilantro, and serve with lemon wedges or a dollop of yogurt if desired.

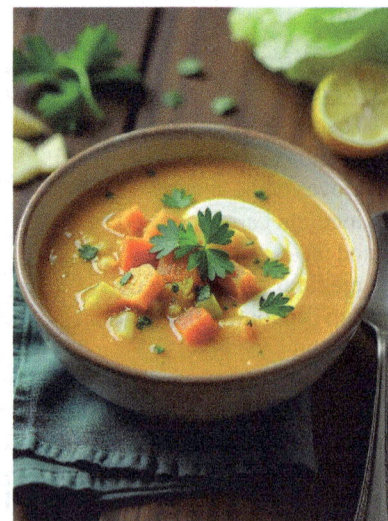

Nutritional Information (per serving):
- **Calories**: 150
- **Protein**: 4g
- **Carbohydrates**: 32g
- **Fiber**: 7g
- **Sugars**: 8g
- **Fats**: 6g
- **Saturated fat**: 1g
- **Cholesterol**: 0mg
- **Sodium**: 500mg (can be adjusted with low-sodium broth)
- **Potassium**: 650mg

CREAMY CAULIFLOWER & LEEK SOUP

Yield: 4 servings • Preparation Time: 10 minutes • Cooking Time: 30 minutes

Ingredients:
For the Soup:
> **11 Tbsp** olive oil
> **2 medium** leeks, cleaned and sliced
> **2 cloves** garlic, minced
> **1 medium** head of cauliflower, chopped
> **1 medium** potato, peeled and diced
> **4 cups** vegetable broth
> **1 cup** coconut milk
> **1/2 tsp** ground turmeric
> **1/4 tsp** ground black pepper
> Salt, to taste
> Fresh lemon juice

Optional Toppings:
> Fresh parsley or chives
> A drizzle of olive oil
> A sprinkle of hemp seeds or chia seeds

Instructions:
1. **Sauté Aromatics**: Heat olive oil in a large pot over medium heat. Add sliced leeks and sauté for 5 minutes until softened. Stir in garlic and cook for 1 minute.
2. **Add Vegetables and Spices**: Add the chopped cauliflower, diced potato, ground turmeric, and ground black pepper. Stir to coat the vegetables with the spices, cooking for about 2-3 minutes to enhance the flavors.
3. **Add Liquids**: Pour in the vegetable broth and bring the mixture to a boil. Once boiling, reduce the heat to low and let the soup simmer, uncovered, for 20-25 minutes or until the cauliflower and potatoes are tender.
4. **Blend the Soup**: Use an immersion blender (or regular blender in batches) to blend the soup until smooth and creamy.
5. **Add Coconut Milk**: After blending, return the soup to the heat and stir in the coconut milk. Let the soup simmer for an additional 5 minutes to allow the flavors to combine.
6. **Taste and Adjust**: Taste the soup and adjust the seasoning with salt, pepper, or a splash of fresh lemon juice for brightness.
7. **Serve**: Ladle into bowls and garnish with parsley, chives, olive oil, or seeds as desired.

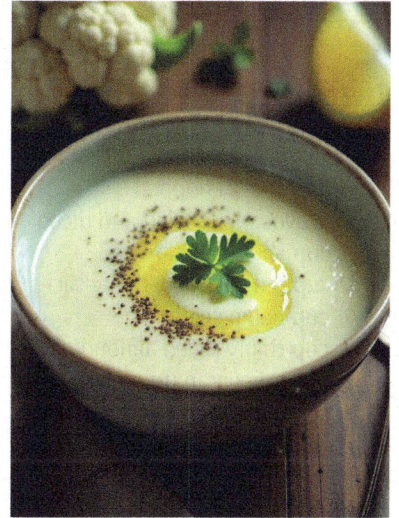

Nutritional Information (per serving):
- **Calories**: 180
- **Protein**: 4g
- **Carbohydrates**: 22g
- **Fiber**: 6g
- **Sugars**: 5g
- **Fats**: 10g
- **Saturated fat**: 7g
- **Cholesterol**: 0mg
- **Sodium**: 300mg (can adjust with low-sodium broth)
- **Potassium**: 650mg

ZUCCHINI & BASIL GREEN SOUP

Yield: 4 servings • Preparation time: 10 minutes • Cooking time: 25 minutes • Total time: 35 minutes

Ingredients:
> **2 medium** zucchinis, chopped
> **1 tablespoon** olive oil
> **1 small** onion, chopped
> **2 garlic cloves**, minced
> **1 cup** vegetable broth
> **1/2 cup** unsweetened coconut milk
> **1/2 cup** fresh basil leaves
> **1/2 teaspoon** ground turmeric
> **1/4 teaspoon** black pepper
> Salt to taste
> **1/2 teaspoon** lemon juice

Optional toppings:
> A few toasted pumpkin seeds for crunch
> A drizzle of extra virgin olive oil
> Fresh basil leaves or microgreens

Instructions:
1. **Sauté the vegetables**: Heat 1 tablespoon of olive oil in a large pot over medium heat. Add the chopped onion and garlic, and sauté for 2-3 minutes until softened and fragrant.
2. **Add zucchini and cook**: Add the chopped zucchinis to the pot and sauté for an additional 5 minutes, stirring occasionally.
3. **Add turmeric and broth**: Sprinkle in the turmeric and black pepper. Stir well to combine, allowing the turmeric to coat the vegetables. Pour in the vegetable broth and bring the mixture to a gentle simmer. Let it cook for 10 minutes, or until the zucchini is soft.
4. **Blend the soup**: Remove the pot from heat and use an immersion blender to purée the soup until smooth. Alternatively, transfer the soup in batches to a countertop blender. If the soup is too thick, you can add a bit more vegetable broth or coconut milk to reach your desired consistency.
5. **Stir in coconut milk and basil**: Return the soup to the stove over low heat. Stir in the coconut milk and fresh basil leaves, and let the soup heat through for another 3-4 minutes.
6. **Season to taste**: Add salt to taste and a squeeze of lemon juice for extra flavor and brightness. If you prefer a creamier texture, feel free to add more coconut milk.
7. **Serve and garnish**: Ladle the soup into bowls, garnish with fresh basil leaves and a drizzle of olive oil. You can also add toasted pumpkin seeds for a crunchy texture.

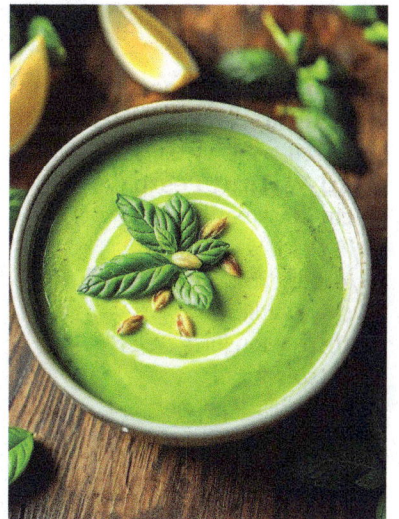

Nutritional Information (per serving):
- **Calories**: 120
- **Protein**: 2g
- **Carbohydrates**: 12g
- **Fats**: 8g
- **Fiber**: 3g
- **Cholesterol**: 0mg
- **Sodium**: 200mg (depending on broth used)
- **Potassium**: 450mg

SALADS & STIR-FRIED VEGETABLES

CRUNCHY KALE SALAD WITH AVOCADO & HEMP SEEDS

Yield: 4 servings • Preparation Time: 15 minutes • Total Time: 15 minutes

Ingredients:
For the Salad:
> **4 cups** fresh kale, washed, stems removed, and chopped
> **1 ripe** avocado, peeled and diced
> **1/2 cup** shredded carrots
> **1/2 cup** red cabbage, thinly sliced
> **1/4 cup** hemp seeds
> **1/4 cup** thinly sliced almonds
> **1/4 cup** pomegranate seeds

For the Lemon-Tahini Dressing:
> **2 tbsp** tahini
> **2 tbsp** fresh lemon juice
> **1 tbsp** apple cider vinegar
> **1 tbsp** extra virgin olive oil
> **1/2 tsp** maple syrup
> **1/4 tsp** turmeric powder
> **1/4 tsp** ground black pepper
> Pinch of Himalayan salt

Instructions:
1. **Massage the Kale**: Place the chopped kale in a large mixing bowl. Add a pinch of salt and gently massage the leaves with your hands for about 2–3 minutes until they soften and darken in color. This step makes the kale easier to digest and enhances its flavor.
2. **Prepare the Dressing**: In a small bowl, whisk together the tahini, lemon juice, apple cider vinegar, olive oil, maple syrup (if using), turmeric, black pepper, and a pinch of salt. Stir until smooth and well combined. Adjust consistency with a little water if needed to make it creamy yet pourable.
3. **Assemble the Salad**: Add the shredded carrots, red cabbage, avocado, hemp seeds, and any optional toppings (sliced almonds, pomegranate seeds) to the massaged kale. Drizzle the dressing over the salad and toss gently to coat everything evenly.
4. **Serve**: Divide the salad into bowls or serve family-style. Enjoy it immediately or let it sit for 10–15 minutes to allow the flavors to meld.

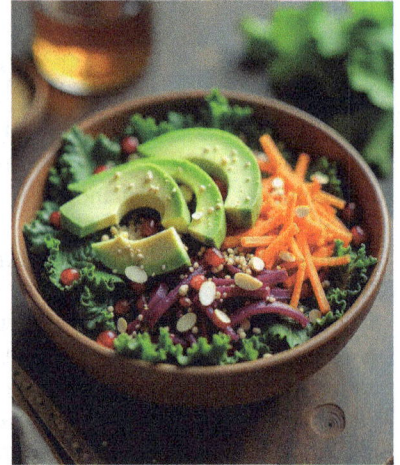

Nutritional Information (per serving):
- **Calories**: 250
- **Protein**: 6g
- **Carbohydrates**: 12g
- **Fats**: 20g
- **Fiber**: 7g
- **Cholesterol**: 0mg
- **Sodium**: 180mg (depending on salt used)
- **Potassium**: 620mg

RAW ZUCCHINI NOODLES WITH PESTO & CHERRY TOMATOES

Yield: 4 servings • Prep Time: 15 minutes • Total Time: 15 minutes

Ingredients:
Zucchini Noodles
> **4 medium** zucchinis, spiralized
> **1 1/2 cups** cherry tomatoes, halved

Basil-Walnut Pesto
> **1 cup** fresh basil leaves
> **1/4 cup** raw walnuts
> **1/4 cup** extra virgin olive oil
> **1 clove** garlic
> **2 tbsp** lemon juice
> **1/4 tsp** sea salt
> **1/4 tsp** black pepper

Optional Add-Ins
> **1 tbsp** nutritional yeast
> Red pepper flakes, to taste, for a spicy kick

Instructions:
1. **Prepare Zucchini Noodles:** Spiralize the zucchinis and set them aside in a large mixing bowl. If you prefer a softer texture, sprinkle a little salt on the noodles and let them sit for 5 minutes, then pat dry.
2. **Make the Pesto:** In a food processor, combine basil, walnuts, olive oil, garlic, lemon juice, sea salt, and black pepper. Blend until smooth and creamy. For a cheesier flavor, add nutritional yeast.
3. **Combine:** Add the pesto to the zucchini noodles and toss until evenly coated. Add halved cherry tomatoes and gently mix.
4. **Serve:** Divide into bowls and top with red pepper flakes if desired.

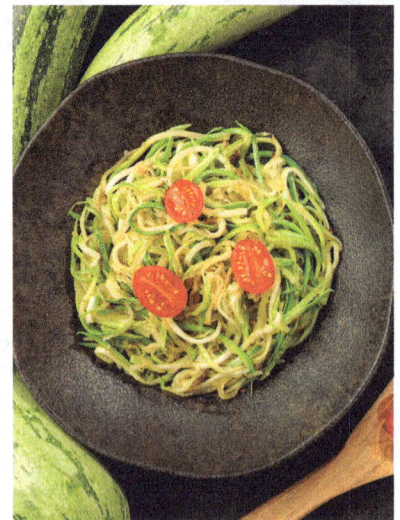

Nutritional Information (per serving):
- **Calories:** 180
- **Protein:** 4g
- **Carbohydrates:** 9g
- **Fats:** 15g
- **Fiber:** 3g
- **Cholesterol:** 0mg
- **Sodium:** 190mg
- **Potassium:** 520mg

COLESLAW WITH PURPLE CABBAGE

Yield: 4 servings • Prep Time: 15 minutes • Total Time: 15 minutes (optional resting time for deeper flavor: 15 minutes)

Ingredients:
Coleslaw
> **2 cups** purple cabbage, thinly sliced
> **1 cup** carrots, shredded
> **1/2 cup** red bell pepper, thinly sliced
> **1/4 cup** fresh parsley, chopped
> **1 tbsp** green onions, thinly sliced (optional)
Dressing
> **3 tbsp** extra virgin olive oil
> **1 tbsp** apple cider vinegar
> **1 tbsp** lemon juice, freshly squeezed
> **1 tsp** honey or maple syrup
> **1/2 tsp** turmeric powder
> **1/4 tsp** ground ginger
> **1/4 tsp** sea salt
> **1/4 tsp** black pepper (for enhanced anti-inflammatory benefits)

Instructions:
1. **Prepare the Vegetables:** Thinly slice the purple cabbage, shred the carrots, and thinly slice the red bell pepper. Place these in a large mixing bowl. Add the chopped parsley and green onions (if using) to the bowl.
2. **Make the Dressing:** In a small bowl, whisk together the olive oil, apple cider vinegar, lemon juice, honey (or maple syrup), turmeric, ground ginger, salt, and black pepper until well combined.
3. **Combine and Toss:** Pour the dressing over the cabbage mixture. Toss gently to ensure the vegetables are evenly coated with the dressing.
4. **Resting Time (Optional):** For best flavor, allow the coleslaw to sit for 15 minutes to let the ingredients marinate. This also softens the cabbage slightly.
5. **Serve and Garnish:** Transfer to a serving dish and garnish with additional parsley or a sprinkle of sesame seeds if desired.

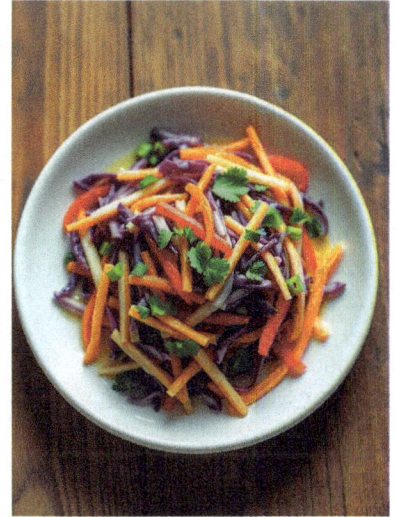

Nutritional Information (per serving):
- **Calories:** 120
- **Protein:** 1g
- **Carbohydrates:** 8g
- **Fats:** 9g
- **Fiber:** 3g
- **Cholesterol:** 0mg
- **Sodium:** 160mg
- **Potassium:** 240mg

SHAVED BRUSSELS SPROUT SALAD WITH LEMON ZEST

Yield: 4 servings • Prep Time: 15 minutes • Total Time: 15 minutes

Ingredients:
> **4 cups** Brussels sprouts, trimmed and thinly shaved
> **1/4 cup** almonds, sliced or slivered
> **1/4 cup** dried cranberries (unsweetened preferred)
> **1/4 cup** extra virgin olive oil
> **2 tbsp** fresh lemon juice
> **1 tsp** lemon zest
> **1 tsp** Dijon mustard
> **1/4 tsp** sea salt
> **1/4 tsp** black pepper
> **Optional: 1 tbsp** fresh parsley, chopped

Instructions:
1. **Prepare Brussels Sprouts:** Trim the ends off the Brussels sprouts, then use a sharp knife, mandoline, or food processor to shave them into thin slices. Transfer to a large salad bowl.
2. **Add Almonds and Cranberries:** Add the sliced almonds and cranberries to the shaved Brussels sprouts.
3. **Make the Dressing:** In a small bowl, whisk together olive oil, lemon juice, lemon zest, Dijon mustard, sea salt, and black pepper until well combined.
4. **Toss Salad with Dressing:** Pour the dressing over the salad and toss thoroughly until all ingredients are evenly coated.
5. **Optional Setting Time (for added flavor):** Allow the salad to sit for 10-15 minutes to allow the flavors to meld, or refrigerate for 30 minutes if you prefer a chilled option.

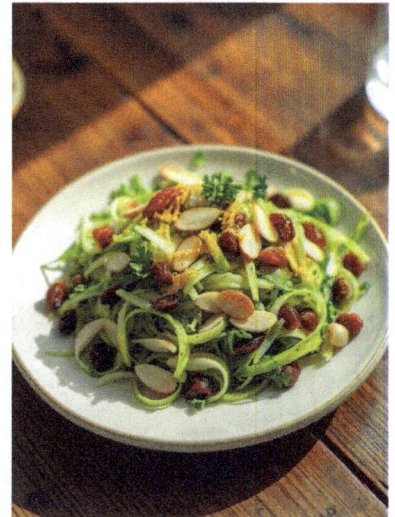

Nutritional Information (per serving):
- **Calories:** 160
- **Protein:** 3 g
- **Carbohydrates:** 8 g
- **Fats:** 13 g
- **Fiber:** 4 g
- **Cholesterol:** 0 mg
- **Sodium:** 90 mg
- **Potassium:** 260 mg

RAINBOW VEGGIE STIR-FRY WITH GINGER SESAME SAUCE

Yield: 4 servings • Prep Time: 15 minutes • Total Time: 25 minutes

Ingredients:

› **1 tbsp** extra virgin olive oil or avocado oil
› **1 cup** red bell pepper, thinly sliced
› **1 cup** carrots, julienned or thinly sliced
› **1 cup** broccoli florets
› **1 cup** zucchini, sliced
› **1/2 cup** purple cabbage, shredded
› **1/2 cup** snow peas, trimmed
› **1/4 cup** green onions, sliced (optional)

Ginger Sesame Sauce:

› **2 tbsp** low-sodium tamari or soy sauce
› **1 tbsp** sesame oil
› **1 tbsp** rice vinegar
› **1 tbsp** fresh ginger, grated
› **1 clove** garlic, minced
› **1 tsp** honey or maple syrup (optional)
› **1 tsp** sesame seeds
› **1/4 tsp** red pepper flakes (optional)

Instructions:

1. **Prepare the Vegetables:** Wash and slice all the vegetables: red bell pepper, carrots, broccoli, zucchini, purple cabbage, and snow peas. Slice the green onions if using.
2. **Make the Ginger Sesame Sauce:** In a small bowl, whisk together the tamari (or soy sauce), sesame oil, rice vinegar, grated ginger, minced garlic, honey or maple syrup (optional), sesame seeds, and red pepper flakes (optional). Set aside.
3. **Cook the Vegetables:** Heat 1 tbsp of olive oil or avocado oil in a large skillet or wok over medium-high heat. Add the carrots, red bell pepper, broccoli, and zucchini. Stir-fry for about 4-5 minutes until tender yet crisp. Add the purple cabbage and snow peas, and stir-fry for another 2-3 minutes until all vegetables are cooked but still retain their vibrant color and crunch.
4. **Toss with Sauce:** Lower the heat to medium and pour the ginger sesame sauce over the cooked vegetables. Stir to coat evenly and heat through for about 1-2 minutes.
5. **Serve:** Transfer the stir-fry to serving bowls. Optionally, top with extra sesame seeds or sliced green onions for garnish.

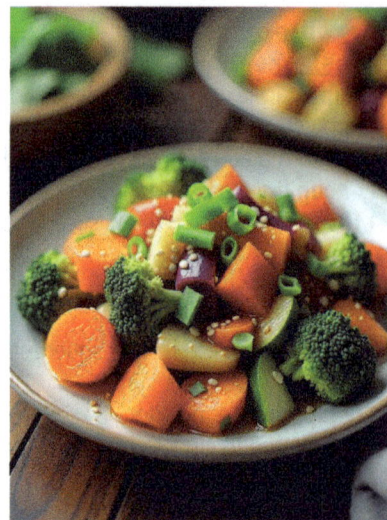

Nutritional Information (per serving):

- **Calories:** 180 kcal
- **Protein:** 4g
- **Carbohydrates:** 20g
- **Fiber:** 6g
- **Sugars:** 6g
- **Fat:** 10g
- **Saturated Fat:** 1g
- **Cholesterol:** 0mg
- **Sodium:** 480mg (depends on the tamari/soy sauce used)
- **Potassium:** 600mg

SAUTÉED SPINACH & GARLIC WITH LEMON ZEST

Yield: 4 servings • Prep Time: 5 minutes • Cooking Time: 10 minutes • Total Time: 15 minutes

Ingredients:

› **1 tbsp** extra virgin olive oil
› **4 cups** fresh spinach, washed and drained
› **3 cloves** garlic, minced
› **1 tsp** fresh lemon zest
› **1 tbsp** fresh lemon juice
› **1/4 tsp** sea salt (or to taste)
› **1/4 tsp** black pepper (or to taste)

Optional:

› **1 tbsp** pine nuts or slivered almonds, toasted
› **1/2 tsp** red pepper flakes for a little heat

Instructions:

1. **Heat the Olive Oil:** Heat 1 tbsp of olive oil in a large skillet over medium heat.
2. **Sauté the Garlic:** Add the minced garlic to the skillet and sauté for 1-2 minutes until fragrant, being careful not to burn it.
3. **Cook the Spinach:** Add the fresh spinach to the skillet in batches, allowing it to wilt down before adding more. Stir occasionally to ensure it cooks evenly, about 3-4 minutes.
4. **Season the Spinach:** Once the spinach is wilted, add the lemon zest, lemon juice, sea salt, and black pepper. Stir well to combine and cook for an additional 1-2 minutes.
5. **Optional Toppings:** If desired, sprinkle with toasted pine nuts or slivered almonds for added texture and nutritional benefits. Optionally, add red pepper flakes for a bit of spice.
6. **Serve:** Transfer the sautéed spinach to a serving dish. Serve warm.

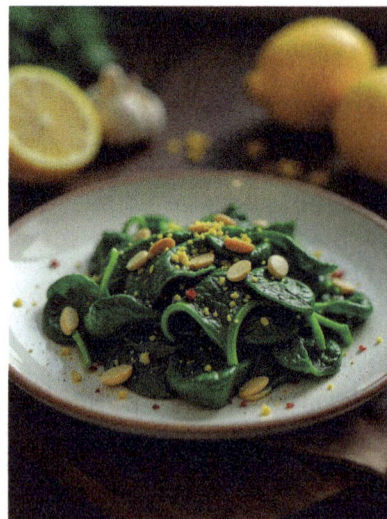

Nutritional Information (per serving):

- **Calories:** 90 kcal
- **Protein:** 3g
- **Carbohydrates:** 6g
- **Fiber:** 4g
- **Sugars:** 1g
- **Fat:** 7g
- **Saturated Fat:** 1g
- **Cholesterol:** 0mg
- **Sodium:** 250mg (depending on salt used)
- **Potassium:** 500mg

9. DESSERTS
FRUIT-BASED DESSERTS

CINNAMON-SPICED APPLE BAKE WITH WALNUTS

Yield: 4 servings • Prep Time: 10 minutes • Total Time: 40 minutes

Ingredients:
> **4 medium** apples (such as Gala, Fuji, or Honeycrisp), cored and sliced
> **1/2 cup** walnuts, chopped
> **1 tbsp** coconut oil, melted
> **1 tbsp** ground cinnamon
> **1/2 tsp** ground ginger
> **1/4 tsp** ground turmeric
> **1 tbsp** maple syrup (optional, for sweetness)
> **1/2 tsp** vanilla extract
> Pinch of sea salt
> **1/4 cup** water

Optional Toppings:
> **1 tbsp** unsweetened shredded coconut
> A dollop of coconut yogurt or plain Greek yogurt
> A drizzle of honey or maple syrup for added sweetness

Instructions:
1. **Preheat the Oven and Prepare Apples:** Preheat the oven to 350°F (175°C). Core and slice the apples into even wedges, then place them in a medium-sized baking dish.
2. **Make the Spiced Mixture:** In a small bowl, combine the cinnamon, ginger, turmeric, and sea salt. Drizzle the melted coconut oil and maple syrup (if using) over the apple slices, then sprinkle the spice mixture over the top. Toss to coat the apples evenly.
3. **Add Walnuts and Water:** Sprinkle the chopped walnuts evenly over the apples. Pour the water into the bottom of the baking dish to help steam the apples as they bake.
4. **Bake the Apples:** Cover the baking dish with aluminum foil and bake for 25 minutes. After 25 minutes, remove the foil and bake for an additional 5–10 minutes, or until the apples are tender and the walnuts are lightly toasted.
5. **Serve:** Once baked, remove from the oven and let cool slightly before serving. Optional: Top with unsweetened shredded coconut, a dollop of coconut yogurt or Greek yogurt, and a drizzle of honey or maple syrup if desired.

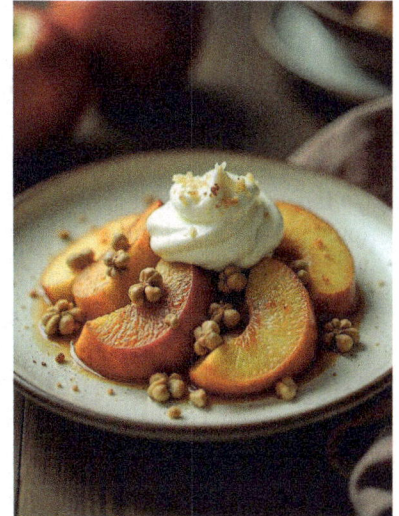

Nutritional Information (per serving):
- **Calories:** 220
- **Protein:** 3 g
- **Carbohydrates:** 28 g
- **Fats:** 14 g
- **Fiber:** 5 g
- **Cholesterol:** 0 mg
- **Sodium:** 60 mg
- **Potassium:** 250 mg

FRESH PINEAPPLE & LIME SORBET

Yield: 4 servings • Prep Time: 15 minutes • Total Time: 3 hours (for freezing)

Ingredients:
> **4 cups** fresh pineapple, peeled and chopped
> **1/4 cup** fresh lime juice (about 2 limes)
> **2 tbsp** honey or maple syrup (optional, for sweetness)
> **1/2 cup** water
> **1/4 tsp** ground turmeric (optional, for added anti-inflammatory benefits)
> Pinch of sea salt

Optional Toppings:
> Fresh mint leaves for garnish
> A sprinkle of shredded coconut for texture
> A drizzle of honey or maple syrup for extra sweetness

Instructions:
1. **Prepare the Pineapple:** Peel and chop the fresh pineapple into small chunks. Place them in a blender or food processor.
2. **Blend the Sorbet Base:** Add the lime juice, honey (if using), water, turmeric (if using), and a pinch of sea salt to the blender with the pineapple. Blend until smooth and creamy, scraping down the sides as needed.
3. **Freeze the Mixture:** Pour the blended mixture into a shallow dish or baking pan. Spread it out evenly and cover with plastic wrap or a lid. Place it in the freezer for about 2–3 hours, or until firm.
4. **Scrape and Serve:** Once the sorbet has frozen, use a fork to scrape the mixture, breaking it into fluffy, ice-crystal-like pieces. Serve immediately, or store in an airtight container in the freezer for up to a week.
5. **Optional Garnishing:** Top with fresh mint leaves, shredded coconut, or a drizzle of honey or maple syrup for added flavor.

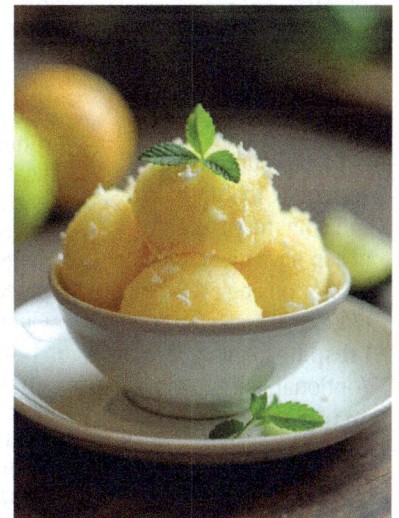

Nutritional Information (per serving):
- **Calories:** 120
- **Protein:** 1 g
- **Carbohydrates:** 31 g
- **Fats:** 0 g
- **Fiber:** 3 g
- **Cholesterol:** 0 mg
- **Sodium:** 5 mg
- **Potassium:** 250 mg

ORANGE & GINGER BAKED FRUIT MEDLEY

Yield: 4 servings • Prep Time: 15 minutes • Total Time: 30 minutes

Ingredients:

> **2 medium** apples, peeled, cored, and sliced
> **2 medium** pears, peeled, cored, and sliced
> **1 cup** fresh pineapple, chopped
> **1/2 cup** orange juice (freshly squeezed)
> **1 tbsp** fresh ginger, grated
> **1 tsp** ground cinnamon
> **1/4 tsp** ground turmeric (optional, for added anti-inflammatory benefits)
> **1 tbsp** maple syrup or honey (optional, for sweetness)
> **1 tbsp** coconut oil (for greasing)

Optional Toppings:

> **2 tbsp** chopped walnuts or almonds for added crunch and healthy fats
> A sprinkle of shredded coconut for texture
> A dollop of Greek yogurt or coconut cream for a creamy finish

Instructions:

1. **Preheat the Oven:** Preheat the oven to 375°F (190°C). Lightly grease a baking dish with coconut oil to prevent the fruit from sticking.
2. **Prepare the Fruit:** Peel, core, and slice the apples and pears. Chop the pineapple into small chunks. Place all the fruit into a large mixing bowl.
3. **Make the Orange & Ginger Sauce:** In a small bowl, combine the orange juice, grated ginger, ground cinnamon, and ground turmeric (if using). Stir well to combine. If you prefer a sweeter medley, add maple syrup or honey to taste.
4. **Toss the Fruit:** Pour the orange-ginger sauce over the fruit in the bowl. Toss gently to coat all the fruit evenly with the sauce.
5. **Bake the Fruit Medley:** Transfer the coated fruit into the prepared baking dish and spread it out evenly. Cover the dish with aluminum foil and bake for 20 minutes. After 20 minutes, remove the foil and bake for an additional 10 minutes, or until the fruit is tender and slightly caramelized.
6. **Optional Garnishing:** After baking, top the fruit medley with chopped walnuts or almonds for added crunch, and sprinkle with shredded coconut for extra texture. For a creamy finish, add a dollop of Greek yogurt or coconut cream on top.

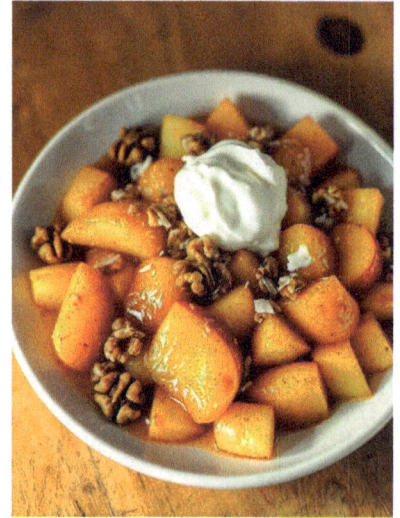

Nutritional Information (per serving):

- **Calories:** 180
- **Protein:** 2 g
- **Carbohydrates:** 45 g
- **Fats:** 5 g
- **Fiber:** 6 g
- **Cholesterol:** 0 mg
- **Sodium:** 15 mg
- **Potassium:** 350 mg

HONEY-GLAZED PEACHES WITH TOASTED ALMONDS

Yield: 4 servings • Prep Time: 10 minutes • Total Time: 20 minutes

Ingredients:

> **4** ripe peaches, halved and pitted
> **2 tbsp** honey (preferably raw, for extra health benefits)
> **1/2 tsp** ground cinnamon
> **1/4 tsp** ground turmeric (optional, for added anti-inflammatory benefits)
> **1 tbsp** olive oil or coconut oil (for grilling or roasting)
> **1/4 cup** sliced almonds
> **1 tbsp** fresh mint, chopped (optional, for garnish)

Optional Toppings:

> A drizzle of additional honey for extra sweetness
> A dollop of Greek yogurt or coconut cream for a creamy finish

Instructions:

1. **Prepare the Peaches:** Cut the peaches in half and remove the pits. If you prefer, you can grill the peaches for a smoky flavor or roast them for a softer texture.
2. **Glaze the Peaches:** In a small bowl, mix together honey, ground cinnamon, and ground turmeric (if using). Stir well until the glaze is smooth and well-combined.
3. **Cook the Peaches:** Heat a grill pan or oven to medium heat. Brush the cut sides of the peach halves with olive oil or coconut oil. Place the peaches, cut side down, on the pan or grill. Cook for 3–4 minutes on each side until grill marks appear or until soft and slightly caramelized. If roasting, preheat the oven to 375°F (190°C) and bake for about 10-12 minutes, or until the peaches are tender.
4. **Toast the Almonds:** While the peaches cook, toast the sliced almonds. Heat a small pan over medium heat, add the almonds, and toast them for 2-3 minutes, stirring frequently to prevent burning. Once golden and fragrant, remove them from the heat.
5. **Glaze and Serve:** Once the peaches are cooked, brush them with the honey glaze. Arrange the peach halves on a serving platter. Sprinkle the toasted almonds over the peaches for a satisfying crunch.
6. **Optional Garnishing:** Garnish with chopped fresh mint for a burst of color and flavor. For extra creaminess, serve with a dollop of Greek yogurt or coconut cream.

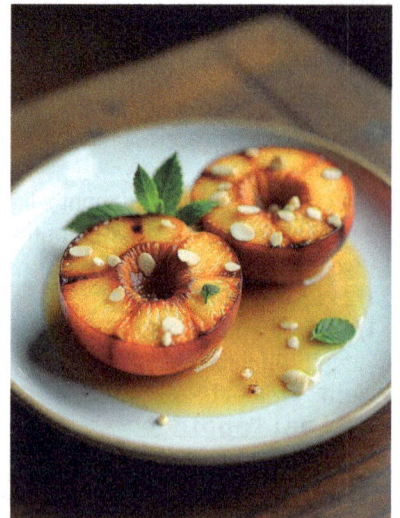

Nutritional Information (per serving):

- **Calories:** 180
- **Protein:** 3 g
- **Carbohydrates:** 28 g
- **Fats:** 8 g
- **Fiber:** 3 g
- **Cholesterol:** 0 mg
- **Sodium:** 2 mg
- **Potassium:** 320 mg

ROASTED FIGS WITH POMEGRANATE SEEDS AND MINT

Yield: 4 servings • Prep Time: 10 minutes • Total Time: 25 minutes

Ingredients:
- **8** ripe figs, halved
- **2 tbsp** olive oil
- **1 tbsp** honey or maple syrup (optional for added sweetness)
- **1/4 tsp** ground cinnamon (optional for extra flavor)
- **1/4 tsp** ground turmeric (optional for extra anti-inflammatory benefits)
- **1/2 cup** pomegranate seeds
- **2 tbsp** fresh mint, chopped
- **1 tbsp** lemon juice (optional, for a tangy kick)

Optional Toppings:
- A drizzle of extra honey or maple syrup
- A sprinkle of crushed pistachios for added crunch and healthy fats
- A few extra mint leaves for garnish

Instructions:
1. **Prepare the Figs:** Preheat the oven to 375°F (190°C). Cut the figs in half and place them on a baking sheet, cut side up.
2. **Season the Figs:** Drizzle the figs with olive oil and honey (if using), then sprinkle with ground cinnamon and turmeric (if using). Use a brush or your hands to evenly coat the figs with the oil and seasoning.
3. **Roast the Figs:** Place the figs in the preheated oven and roast for about 12-15 minutes, or until they are soft and caramelized. Keep an eye on them to ensure they don't burn.
4. **Prepare the Toppings:** While the figs are roasting, prepare the pomegranate seeds by cutting open the pomegranate and removing the seeds. Chop the fresh mint and set both ingredients aside.
5. **Assemble the Dish:** Once the figs are roasted and slightly cooled, arrange them on a serving platter. Sprinkle the pomegranate seeds evenly over the figs, followed by the chopped mint.
6. **Optional Garnishing:** If desired, drizzle a bit of extra honey or maple syrup over the figs for additional sweetness. Garnish with a few extra mint leaves or a sprinkle of crushed pistachios for added flavor and crunch.

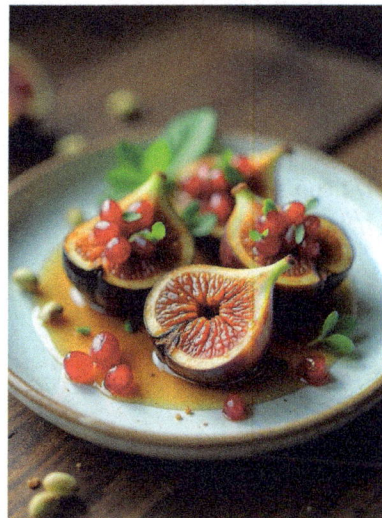

Nutritional Information (per serving):
- **Calories:** 170
- **Protein:** 2 g
- **Carbohydrates:** 30 g
- **Fats:** 7 g
- **Fiber:** 5 g
- **Cholesterol:** 0 mg
- **Sodium:** 3 mg
- **Potassium:** 375 mg

PEAR & BLUEBERRY CRISP WITH ALMOND FLOUR TOPPING

Yield: 6 servings • Prep Time: 15 minutes • Total Time: 45 minutes

Ingredients For the Fruit Filling:
- **4** ripe pears, peeled, cored, and sliced
- **1 cup** fresh or frozen blueberries
- **1 tbsp** fresh lemon juice
- **1 tbsp** maple syrup (optional, for extra sweetness)
- **1 tsp** ground cinnamon
- **1/4 tsp** ground ginger (optional, for extra anti-inflammatory benefits)
- **1 tbsp** arrowroot powder or cornstarch (optional, for thickening)

For the Almond Flour Topping:
- **1 cup** almond flour
- **1/4 cup** rolled oats (optional, for added texture)
- **1/4 cup** chopped walnuts (optional, for added crunch and anti-inflammatory omega-3s)
- **2 tbsp** coconut oil, melted
- **2 tbsp** maple syrup or honey
- **1/2 tsp** ground cinnamon
- **1/4 tsp** ground ginger
- **1/8 tsp** sea salt

Optional Toppings:
- A dollop of coconut whipped cream or Greek yogurt
- A sprinkle of chia seeds for added omega-3s
- Fresh mint leaves for garnish

Instructions:
1. **Preheat Oven and Prepare Baking Dish:** Preheat your oven to 350°F (175°C). Grease a 9x9-inch baking dish with a little coconut oil or line it with parchment paper for easy cleanup.
2. **Prepare the Fruit Filling:** In a large bowl, toss the pear slices, blueberries, lemon juice, maple syrup (if using), ground cinnamon, and ground ginger. If you'd like a thicker filling, sprinkle the arrowroot powder or cornstarch over the fruit mixture and toss to coat evenly. Transfer the fruit mixture to the prepared baking dish.
3. **Make the Almond Flour Topping:** In a separate bowl, combine the almond flour, rolled oats (if using), walnuts (if using), melted coconut oil, maple syrup or honey, ground cinnamon, ground ginger, and sea salt. Stir until the mixture is well combined and crumbly.
4. **Assemble the Crisp:** Evenly spread the almond flour topping over the prepared fruit mixture in the baking dish.
5. **Bake the Crisp:** Bake the crisp in the preheated oven for 30-35 minutes, or until the fruit is bubbling and the topping is golden brown.
6. **Cool and Serve:** Let the crisp cool for about 10 minutes before serving. Optionally, top with a dollop of coconut whipped cream, Greek yogurt, chia seeds, or fresh mint leaves.

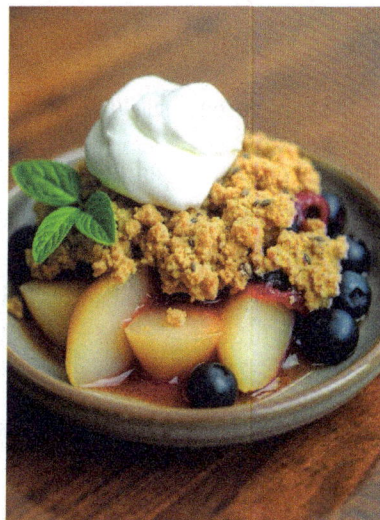

Nutritional Information (per serving):
- **Calories:** 250
- **Protein:** 4 g
- **Carbohydrates:** 30 g
- **Fats:** 14 g
- **Fiber:** 6 g
- **Cholesterol:** 0 mg
- **Sodium:** 70 mg
- **Potassium:** 350 mg

ANTI-INFLAMMATORY TREATS

NO-BAKE TURMERIC & GINGER COCONUT BALLS

Yield: 12-14 balls • Prep Time: 15 minutes • Chilling Time: 30 minutes • Total Time: 45 minutes

Ingredients:
> **1 cup** unsweetened shredded coconut
> **1/2 cup** almond flour
> **1/4 cup** raw honey or maple syrup (optional, for sweetness)
> **1 tbsp** coconut oil (melted)
> **1 tsp** ground turmeric
> **1/2 tsp** ground ginger
> **1/4 tsp** cinnamon (optional, for extra flavor)
> **1/4 tsp** vanilla extract
> Pinch of sea salt
> **1 tbsp** chia seeds or flaxseed (optional, for added fiber)
> **1-2 tbsp** water (if needed, to adjust consistency)

Optional Toppings:
> Additional shredded coconut for rolling
> Chopped almonds or walnuts for a crunchy coating

Instructions:
1. **Combine dry ingredients:** In a medium bowl, mix together the shredded coconut, almond flour, ground turmeric, ground ginger, cinnamon (if using), and a pinch of sea salt.
2. **Add wet ingredients:** Stir in the raw honey or maple syrup, melted coconut oil, and vanilla extract. Mix until everything is well combined, and a sticky dough begins to form.
3. **Adjust consistency:** If the mixture seems too dry, add 1-2 tbsp of water, one tablespoon at a time, until the dough holds together but isn't too wet.
4. **Shape the balls:** Using about 1 tablespoon of the mixture at a time, roll the dough into balls with your hands. You should get about 12-14 balls, depending on the size.
5. **Optional coating:** If desired, roll each ball in extra shredded coconut, chopped nuts (like almonds or walnuts), or a little more cinnamon for added texture and flavor.
6. **Chill:** Place the balls on a plate lined with parchment paper and refrigerate for at least 30 minutes to firm up.
7. **Serve and enjoy:** Once the balls are chilled and firm, they are ready to be enjoyed as a healthy, anti-inflammatory snack.

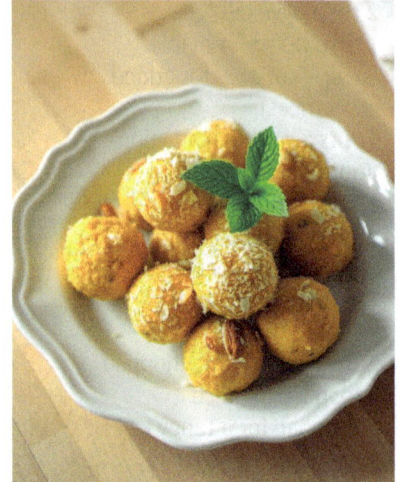

Nutritional Information (per serving, 1 ball):
- **Calories:** 120
- **Protein:** 2 g
- **Carbohydrates:** 10 g
- **Fats:** 8 g
- **Fiber:** 2 g
- **Cholesterol:** 0 mg
- **Sodium:** 10 mg
- **Potassium:** 90 mg

GOLDEN MILK POPSICLES WITH COCONUT CREAM

Yield: 6 popsicles • Prep Time: 10 minutes • Passive Freezing Time: 4 hours • Total Time: 4 hours 10 minutes

Ingredients:
> **1 1/2 cups** coconut milk (full-fat for creaminess)
> **1/2 cup** coconut cream
> **1 tsp** ground turmeric
> **1/2 tsp** ground ginger
> **1/2 tsp** cinnamon
> **1/8 tsp** black pepper (enhances turmeric absorption)
> **2 tbsp** honey or maple syrup (optional, for sweetness)
> **1/2 tsp** vanilla extract (optional for added flavor)

Optional Add-Ins:
> **1 tbsp** chia seeds (for added fiber and omega-3s)
> **1/4 tsp** ground cardamom (for a warming, aromatic flavor)

Instructions:
1. **Combine ingredients:**
   In a medium bowl, whisk together the coconut milk, coconut cream, turmeric, ginger, cinnamon, black pepper, honey or maple syrup (if using), and vanilla extract. Stir well to ensure the spices are fully mixed in.
2. **Add optional ingredients:** If using chia seeds or cardamom, stir them in. Let the mixture sit for a few minutes to allow the chia seeds to hydrate slightly.
3. **Pour into molds:** Carefully pour the mixture into popsicle molds, leaving a little space at the top to allow for expansion when freezing.
4. **Freeze:** Place popsicle sticks into the molds and freeze for at least 4 hours, or until solid.
5. **Serve:** Once frozen, run the molds under warm water for a few seconds to loosen, then remove the popsicles from the molds. Serve immediately.

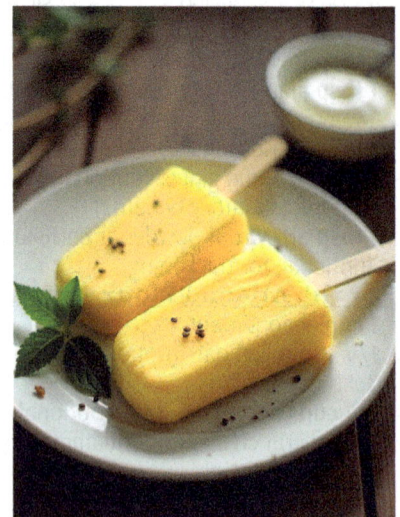

Nutritional Information (per serving, 1 popsicle):
- **Calories:** 140
- **Protein:** 1 g
- **Carbohydrates:** 4 g
- **Fats:** 13 g
- **Fiber:** 1 g
- **Cholesterol:** 0 mg
- **Sodium:** 8 mg
- **Potassium:** 160 mg

CASHEW & COCONUT CHIA PUDDING WITH RASPBERRIES

Yield: 4 servings • Prep Time: 10 minutes • Passive Setting Time: 4 hours or overnight • Total Time: 4 hours 10 minutes

Ingredients:
> **1 1/2 cups** unsweetened coconut milk
> **1/4 cup** chia seeds
> **2 tbsp** cashew butter (or 1/4 cup raw cashews, soaked and blended)
> **1 tbsp** maple syrup or honey (optional for added sweetness)
> **1/2 tsp** vanilla extract (optional)
> **1/4 cup** fresh raspberries, plus extra for topping

Optional Add-Ins:
> **1/2 tsp** ground cinnamon (for anti-inflammatory benefits)
> **1 tbsp** shredded coconut (for extra texture and flavor)

Instructions:
1. **Prepare the Base:** In a mixing bowl, whisk together coconut milk, cashew butter, chia seeds, maple syrup (if using), and vanilla extract until smooth and well-combined.
2. **Add Raspberries:** Lightly mash 1/4 cup raspberries and stir them into the chia mixture to distribute flavor and color.
3. **Set and Chill:** Cover the bowl or divide into individual jars, and refrigerate for at least 4 hours, or overnight, until the chia seeds have gelled and the pudding has thickened.
4. **Serve and Garnish:** Once set, stir the pudding. Top with fresh raspberries, shredded coconut, or a sprinkle of cinnamon, if desired.

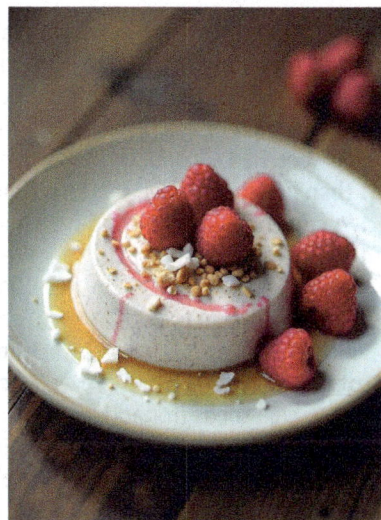

Nutritional Information (per serving):
- **Calories**: ~210 kcal
- **Fiber**: 8g
- **Protein**: 5g
- **Cholesterol**: 0mg
- **Carbohydrates**: 16g
- **Sodium**: 30mg
- **Fats**: 15g
- **Potassium**: 300mg

LEMON & GINGER BARS

Yield: 8 servings • Prep Time: 15 minutes • Cooking Time: 20 minutes • Passive Cooling Time: 30 minutes • Total Time: 1 hour 5 minutes

Ingredients:
Base Layer:
> **1 cup** almond flour
> **1/4 cup** coconut flour
> **1/4 cup** coconut oil, melted
> **2 tbsp** maple syrup or honey
> **1/4 tsp** sea salt

Lemon & Ginger Layer:
> **2 large** eggs
> **1/3 cup** fresh lemon juice (about 2 lemons)
> **1 tbsp** lemon zest
> **2 tbsp** maple syrup or honey
> **1 tsp** freshly grated ginger
> **1/2 tsp** ground turmeric
> **1/4 cup** coconut flour

Optional Toppings:
> **1 tbsp** shredded coconut
> **1 tsp** chia seeds

Instructions:
1. **Preheat and Prepare the Pan:** Preheat the oven to 350°F (175°C). Line an 8x8-inch baking dish with parchment paper, allowing the edges to hang over for easy removal.
2. **Make the Base Layer:** In a medium bowl, mix the almond flour, coconut flour, melted coconut oil, maple syrup, and sea salt until well combined. Press this mixture firmly and evenly into the bottom of the prepared baking dish. Bake for 10 minutes, then remove from the oven and let it cool slightly.
3. **Prepare the Lemon & Ginger Layer:** In a separate bowl, whisk the eggs until light and frothy. Add the lemon juice, lemon zest, maple syrup, grated ginger, and ground turmeric. Whisk well, then sift in the coconut flour, stirring until the mixture is smooth.
4. **Assemble and Bake:** Pour the lemon-ginger mixture over the pre-baked base layer, spreading evenly. Return the dish to the oven and bake for an additional 15–20 minutes, or until the lemon layer is set and lightly golden.
5. **Cool and Set:** Remove the dish from the oven and let it cool completely in the pan. Once cool, refrigerate for at least 30 minutes to fully set.
6. **Serve and Garnish:** Once chilled, lift the bars out using the parchment overhang, slice into 8 squares, and garnish with shredded coconut and chia seeds if desired.

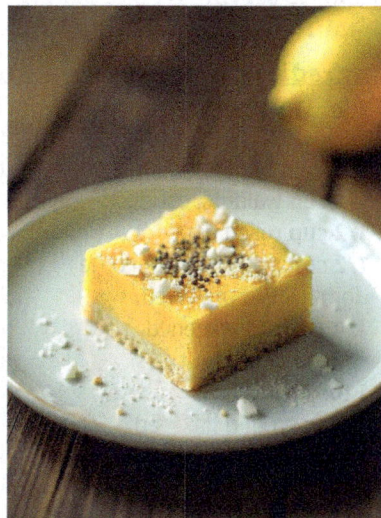

Nutritional Information (per serving):
- **Calories**: ~180 kcal
- **Cholesterol**: 30mg
- **Protein**: 4g
- **Sodium**: 60mg
- **Carbohydrates**: 13g
- **Potassium**: 70mg
- **Fats**: 14g
- **Fiber**: 3g

MATCHA & COCONUT BLISS BALLS WITH ALMONDS

Yield: 12 servings (1 ball per serving) • Prep Time: 10 minutes • Passive Setting Time: 20–30 minutes (refrigeration)
Total Time: 30–40 minutes

Ingredients:
Base Ingredients:
> **1 cup** raw almonds
> **1/2 cup** shredded unsweetened coconut
> **1 tbsp** matcha powder
> **1/4 cup** coconut oil, melted
> **1/4 cup** maple syrup or honey
> **1/2 tsp** vanilla extract
> Pinch of salt

Optional Add-Ins:
> **1 tbsp** chia seeds (for added fiber and omega-3s)
> 1 tbsp hemp seeds (for additional protein and omega-3s)
> **1 tbsp** cacao nibs (for a chocolatey crunch)

Instructions:
1. **Prepare the Almonds and Coconut**: In a food processor, pulse the almonds and shredded coconut until they are finely ground but not turned into a paste. Aim for a coarse, sandy texture.
2. **Add Remaining Ingredients**: Add the matcha powder, melted coconut oil, maple syrup, vanilla extract, and salt to the food processor. Pulse again until all ingredients are well combined and the mixture sticks together when pressed.
3. **Incorporate Optional Add-Ins**: If using, add chia seeds, hemp seeds, or cacao nibs to the mixture and pulse briefly to mix them in without over-processing.
4. **Form the Balls**: Scoop about 1 tbsp of the mixture and roll it between your hands to form a ball. Repeat with the remaining mixture to make about 12 bliss balls.
5. **Chill**: Place the bliss balls in the refrigerator for 20–30 minutes to set. This helps them hold their shape.
6. **Serve**: Enjoy immediately or store in an airtight container in the refrigerator for up to one week.

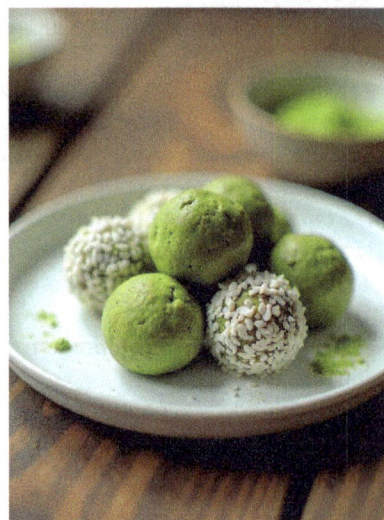

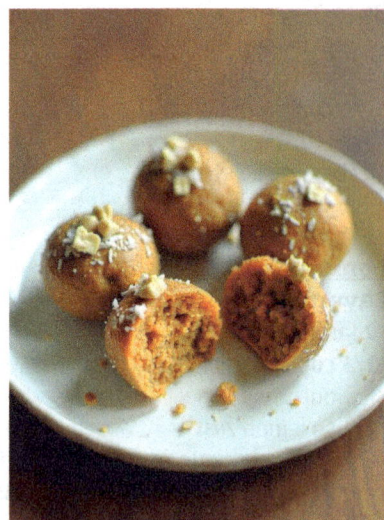

Nutritional Information (per serving – 1 bliss ball):
- **Calories**: ~110 kcal
- **Protein**: 2g
- **Carbohydrates**: 5g
- **Fats**: 9g
- **Fiber**: 2g
- **Cholesterol**: 0mg
- **Sodium**: 5mg
- **Potassium**: 75mg

CARROT CAKE BITES WITH CINNAMON AND WALNUTS

Yield: 12 servings (1 bite per serving) • Prep Time: 15 minutes • Passive Setting Time: 30 minutes (refrigeration) •
Total Time: 45 minutes

Ingredients
Base Ingredients:
> **1 cup** grated carrot (about 2 medium carrots)
> **1/2 cup** walnuts, chopped
> **1/2 cup** rolled oats
> **1/2 cup** pitted Medjool dates (or raisins if preferred)
> **1/4 cup** unsweetened shredded coconut
> **1 tbsp** chia seeds
> **1 tbsp** ground flaxseed
> **1 tsp** ground cinnamon
> **1/4 tsp** ground ginger
> **1/4 tsp** nutmeg
> Pinch of salt

Optional Add-Ins:
> **1/2 tsp** vanilla extract (for added flavor)
> **1 tbsp** almond butter (for extra creaminess)

Instructions
1. **Prepare Ingredients**: Place the grated carrot on a clean towel and squeeze out excess moisture. This prevents the bites from becoming too wet.
2. **Blend Base Ingredients**: In a food processor, combine the oats, dates, walnuts, shredded coconut, chia seeds, ground flaxseed, cinnamon, ginger, nutmeg, and salt. Pulse until the mixture is well combined and sticky. The oats and walnuts should be finely chopped but not completely smooth.
3. **Add Carrots and Optional Ingredients**: Add the grated carrot (and almond butter or vanilla if using) to the food processor and pulse again until everything is well incorporated. The mixture should hold together when pressed. If it's too dry, add a little more almond butter or a few drops of water.
4. **Form the Bites**: Scoop about 1 tbsp of the mixture and roll it into a ball between your hands. Repeat with the remaining mixture to make about 12 bites.
5. **Chill**: Place the bites on a plate or tray and refrigerate for 30 minutes to set. This helps them firm up and enhances the flavors.
6. **Serve**: Enjoy immediately, or store in an airtight container in the refrigerator for up to one week.

Nutritional Information (per serving – 1 bite)
- **Calories**: ~90 kcal
- **Protein**: 2g
- **Carbohydrates**: 12g
- **Fats**: 4g
- **Fiber**: 2g
- **Cholesterol**: 0mg
- **Sodium**: 10mg
- **Potassium**: 120mg

MEAL PLAN

Day	Breakfast	Lunch	Dinner	Dessert
1	Matcha Green Smoothie with Spinach and Mango (12)	Lemon & Herb Chicken Skewers with Cucumber Salad (41), Lemon & Herb Quinoa with Roasted Vegetables (30)	Ginger & Lime Grilled Shrimp Skewers (36), Arugula, Apple & Pecan Salad with Lemon Vinaigrette (24)	Cinnamon-Spiced Apple Bake with Walnuts (63)
2	Apple-Cinnamon Overnight Oats with Walnuts (15)	Lemon-Rosemary Grilled Lamb Chops (48), Wild Rice Pilaf with Cranberries and Pecans (32)	Lemon-Pepper Baked Cod with Fresh Parsley (36), Crunchy Kale Salad with Avocado & Hemp Seeds (60)	Honey-Glazed Peaches with Toasted Almonds (64)
3	Orange & Carrot Sunrise Smoothie with Turmeric (13)	Turkey & Sweet Potato Chili (45), Coconut & Ginger Millet with Carrots (31)	Miso-Marinated Sea Bass with Bok Choy (38), Shaved Brussels Sprout Salad with Lemon Zest (61)	Cashew & Coconut Chia Pudding with Raspberries (67)
4	Buckwheat & Berry Porridge with Coconut Milk (15)	Grilled Pork Chops with Fresh Herbs (50), Turmeric-Spiced Bulgur with Mixed Herbs (32)	Moroccan-Spiced Fish Stew with Saffron (39), Mixed Greens with Golden Beets and Pomegranate Seeds (25)	Fresh Pineapple & Lime Sorbet (63)
5	Anti-Inflammatory Blueberry & Kale Smoothie (12)	Chicken & Sweet Potato Curry with Coconut (44), Anti-Inflammatory Barley & Mushroom Risotto (30)	Moroccan-Spiced Fish Stew with Saffron (39), Endive & Walnut Salad with Pomegranate Dressing (26)	Roasted Figs with Pomegranate Seeds and Mint (65)
6	Chia & Hemp Seed Pudding with Fresh Mango (17)	Beef & Veggie Stir-Fry with Ginger (48), Golden Farro with Sweet Potatoes & Sage (31)	Baked Salmon with Sweet Potato & Fennel (38), Watercress & Pear Salad with Hazelnuts (26)	Orange & Ginger Baked Fruit Medley (64)
7	Blackberry & Banana Oat Smoothie (14)	Roasted Herb Chicken with Root Vegetables (47), Chickpea Pasta with Spinach & Walnut Pesto (33)	Cucumber & Dill Salmon Ceviche (37), Millet & Zucchini Salad with Fresh Basil (28)	Anti-Inflammatory Lemon & Ginger Bars (67)

Shopping List 1-7 Days

Fruits and Vegetables

◊ Mango – 3

◊ Green apples – 2

◊ Fresh peaches – 2

◊ Fresh oranges – 3

◊ Raspberries – 1 cup

◊ Fresh blueberries – 1 cup

◊ Fresh pineapple – 1 medium

◊ Fresh bananas – 2

◊ Fresh pears – 2

◊ Fresh figs – 4

◊ Lemons – 4

◊ Limes – 2

◊ Fresh spinach – 3 cups

◊ Carrots – 6 medium

◊ Zucchini – 3 medium

◊ Kale – 4 cups

◊ Arugula – 2 cups

◊ Fresh brussels sprouts – 1 lb

◊ Sweet potatoes – 4 medium

◊ Butternut squash – 1 small

◊ Mixed greens – 2 cups

◊ Golden beets – 2

◊ Fresh fennel – 1 bulb

◊ Fresh parsley,thyme, basil,dill,cilantro,mint ,rosemary

◊ Bok choy – 1 head

◊ Cucumber – 2 medium

Meat & Seafood

◊ Chicken breasts (for skewers) – 2 pieces (about 1 lb)

◊ Shrimp – 1 lb

◊ Lamb chops – 2 pieces (about 1 lb)

◊ Cod fillets – 2 pieces (about 1 lb)

◊ Sea bass fillets – 2 pieces (about 1 lb)

◊ Halibut fillets – 2 pieces (about 1 lb)

◊ Salmon fillets – 2 pieces (about 1 lb)

◊ Pork chops – 2 pieces (about 1 lb)

◊ Ground turkey – 1 lb

Day	Breakfast	Lunch	Dinner	Dessert
8	Spinach & Green Apple Immunity Booster Smoothie (13)	Cilantro-Ginger Marinated Chicken Breast (42), Wild Rice Pilaf with Cranberries and Pecans (32)	Grilled Swordfish with Olive & Tomato Relish (40), Arugula, Apple & Pecan Salad with Lemon Vinaigrette (24)	Pear & Blueberry Crisp with Almond Flour Topping (65)
9	Oatmeal with Turmeric, Cinnamon & Apples (17)	Pork Tenderloin with Apple-Mustard Glaze (49), Lemon & Herb Quinoa with Roasted Vegetables (30)	Anti-Inflammatory Steamed Mussels with Garlic (37), Crunchy Kale Salad with Avocado & Hemp Seeds (60)	Golden Milk Popsicles with Coconut Cream (66)
10	Avocado & Kiwi Anti-Inflammatory Smoothie (14)	Braised Chicken Thighs with Ginger & Carrots (45), Chickpea Pasta with Spinach & Walnut Pesto (33)	Broiled Tuna Steaks with Mango Salsa (39), Shaved Brussels Sprout Salad with Lemon Zest (61)	Honey-Glazed Peaches with Toasted Almonds (64)
11	Quinoa Breakfast Bowl with Cherries and Hemp Seeds (16)	Lean Beef Skewers with Bell Peppers (49), Golden Farro with Sweet Potatoes & Sage (31)	Lemon-Pepper Baked Cod with Fresh Parsley (36), Watercress & Pear Salad with Hazelnuts (26)	Anti-Inflammatory Lemon & Ginger Bars (67)
12	Anti-Inflammatory Golden Millet Porridge with Figs (16)	Coconut-Curry Turkey Meatballs (46), Turmeric-Spiced Bulgur with Mixed Herbs (32)	Herb-Crusted Halibut with Lemon (39), Mixed Greens with Golden Beets and Pomegranate Seeds (25)	Matcha & Coconut Bliss Balls with Almonds (68)
13	Orange & Carrot Sunrise Smoothie with Turmeric (13)	Turkey & Sweet Potato Chili (45), Zucchini Noodles with Basil, Tomato & Garlic (33)	Miso-Marinated Sea Bass with Bok Choy (38), Romaine, Cucumber & Dill Salad with Olive Oil (25)	Cinnamon-Spiced Apple Bake with Walnuts (63)
14	Chia & Hemp Seed Pudding with Fresh Mango (17)	Honey & Turmeric Pork Meatballs (52), Anti-Inflammatory Barley & Mushroom Risotto (30)	Moroccan-Spiced Fish Stew with Saffron (39), Endive & Walnut Salad with Pomegranate Dressing (26)	No-Bake Turmeric & Ginger Coconut Balls (66)

Shopping List 8- 14 Days

Fruits and Vegetables

◊ Green apples – 3

◊ Pears – 3

◊ Mango – 2

◊ Peaches – 2

◊ Fresh cherries – 1/2 cup

◊ Kiwi – 2

◊ Fresh figs – 4

◊ Oranges – 1

◊ Lemons – 6

◊ Fresh pomegranate) – 1

◊ Bananas – 1 (optional for smoothies)

◊ Fresh spinach – 3 cups

◊ Fresh kale – 4 cups

◊ Carrots – 6 medium

◊ Zucchini – 3 medium

◊ Sweet potatoes – 4 medium

◊ Bell peppers – 3 medium

◊ Brussels sprouts – 1 lb

◊ Romaine lettuce – 2 cups

◊ Cucumber – 1 medium

◊ Endive – 2 heads

◊ Watercress – 2 cups

◊ Fresh ginger – 5-inch piece

◊ Fresh garlic – 4 cloves

◊ Fresh parsley,thyme, basil,dill,cilantro,mint

◊ Golden beets – 2

◊ Fresh mushrooms – 1 cup

◊ Fresh onions – 2 small

◊ Fresh avocado – 2

◊ Fresh tomatoes – 2 medium

◊ Shaved brussels sprouts – 1 lb

◊ Fresh bok choy – 2 heads

Meat & Seafood

◊ Chicken breasts – 2 (about 1 lb)

◊ Chicken thighs – 4 pieces (about 1 lb)

◊ Lean beef (for skewers) – 1 lb

◊ Pork tenderloin – 1 lb

◊ Ground turkey – 2 lb

◊ Ground pork – 1 lb

◊ Fresh swordfish steaks – 2 (about 1 lb)

◊ Fresh tuna steaks – 2 pieces (about 1 lb)

◊ Cod fillets – 2 pieces (about 1 lb)

◊ Halibut fillets – 2 pieces (about 1 lb)

◊ Sea bass fillets – 2 pieces (about 1 lb)

◊ Fresh mussels – 1 lb

◊ White fish fillets (for Moroccan-spiced stew) – 1 lb

Day	Breakfast	Lunch	Dinner	Dessert
15	Anti-Inflammatory Blueberry & Kale Smoothie (12)	Braised Beef with Carrots and Celery (51), Coconut & Ginger Millet with Carrots (31)	Baked Salmon with Sweet Potato & Fennel (38), Mixed Greens with Golden Beets and Pomegranate Seeds (25)	Orange & Ginger Baked Fruit Medley (64)
16	Apple-Cinnamon Overnight Oats with Walnuts (15)	Lemon & Herb Chicken Skewers with Cucumber Salad (41), Wild Rice & Blueberry Salad with Spinach (27)	Grilled Swordfish with Olive & Tomato Relish (40), Crunchy Kale Salad with Avocado & Hemp Seeds (60)	Cashew & Coconut Chia Pudding with Raspberries (67)
17	Matcha Green Smoothie with Spinach and Mango (12)	Spiced Beef & Lentil Casserole (53), Quinoa & Roasted Butternut Squash Salad (28)	White Fish & Sweet Potato Coconut Stew (41), Shaved Brussels Sprout Salad with Lemon Zest (61)	Fresh Pineapple & Lime Sorbet (63)
18	Buckwheat & Berry Porridge with Coconut Milk (15)	Basil & Spinach Pesto Chicken (43), Lentil Pasta with Roasted Tomato Sauce (35)	Anti-Inflammatory Steamed Mussels with Garlic (37), Romaine, Cucumber & Dill Salad with Olive Oil (25)	Roasted Figs with Pomegranate Seeds and Mint (65)
19	Blackberry & Banana Oat Smoothie (14)	Roasted Venison with Garlic & Thyme (50), Turmeric-Spiced Bulgur with Mixed Herbs (32)	Moroccan-Spiced Fish Stew with Saffron (39), Watercress & Pear Salad with Hazelnuts (26)	Golden Milk Popsicles with Coconut Cream (66)
20	Avocado & Kiwi Anti-Inflammatory Smoothie (14)	Coconut-Curry Turkey Meatballs (46), Quinoa Pasta Primavera with Artichoke Hearts (34)	Miso-Marinated Sea Bass with Bok Choy (38), Endive & Walnut Salad with Pomegranate Dressing (26)	No-Bake Turmeric & Ginger Coconut Balls (66)
21	Quinoa Breakfast Bowl with Cherries and Hemp Seeds (16)	Grilled Pork Chops with Fresh Herbs (50), Golden Farro with Sweet Potatoes & Sage (31)	Ginger & Lime Grilled Shrimp Skewers (36), Romaine, Cucumber & Dill Salad with Olive Oil (25)	Anti-Inflammatory Lemon & Ginger Bars (67)

Shopping List 15- 21 Days

Fruits and Vegetables

◊ Blueberries – 2 cups
◊ Fresh mango – 2
◊ Fresh pineapple – 1 medium
◊ Fresh bananas – 2
◊ Green apples – 2
◊ Oranges – 3
◊ Lemons – 4
◊ Raspberries – 1 cup
◊ Fresh figs – 4
◊ Pears – 2
◊ Fresh cherries – 1/2 cup
◊ Fresh limes – 2
◊ Pomegranate (or pomegranate seeds) – 1
◊ Fresh kale – 4 cups

◊ Carrots – 6 medium
◊ Celery – 2 stalks
◊ Sweet potatoes – 4 medium
◊ Fennel – 1 bulb
◊ Mixed greens – 4 cups
◊ Golden beets – 2
◊ Butternut squash – 1 small
◊ Romaine lettuce – 2 cups
◊ Cucumber – 2 medium
◊ Brussels sprouts – 1 lb
◊ Fresh spinach – 3 cups
◊ Fresh parsley, thyme, basil, dill, cilantro, mint
◊ Artichoke hearts (canned or jarred) – 1/2 cup

Meat & Seafood

◊ Beef stew meat (for braised beef) – 1 lb
◊ Chicken breast (for skewers) – 2 pieces (about 1 lb)
◊ Swordfish steaks – 2 pieces (about 1 lb)
◊ Salmon fillets – 2 pieces (about 1 lb)
◊ Ground turkey (for meatballs) – 1 lb
◊ White fish fillets (for stew) – 1 lb
◊ Halibut fillets – 2 pieces (about 1 lb)
◊ Sea bass fillets – 2 pieces (about 1 lb)
◊ Shrimp (for skewers) – 1 lb
◊ Venison (or other lean meat for roasting) – 1 lb
◊ Pork chops – 2 pieces (about 1 lb)

Day	Breakfast	Lunch	Dinner	Dessert
22	Spinach & Green Apple Immunity Booster Smoothie (13)	Honey & Turmeric Pork Meatballs (52), Wild Rice Pilaf with Cranberries and Pecans (32)	Grilled Swordfish with Olive & Tomato Relish (40), Arugula, Apple & Pecan Salad with Lemon Vinaigrette (24)	Pear & Blueberry Crisp with Almond Flour Topping (65)
23	Chia & Hemp Seed Pudding with Fresh Mango (17)	Braised Chicken Thighs with Ginger & Carrots (45), Coconut & Ginger Millet with Carrots (31)	Lemon-Pepper Baked Cod with Fresh Parsley (36), Shaved Brussels Sprout Salad with Lemon Zest (61)	Fresh Pineapple & Lime Sorbet (63)
24	Anti-Inflammatory Golden Millet Porridge with Figs (16)	Lemon-Rosemary Grilled Lamb Chops (48), Quinoa & Roasted Butternut Squash Salad (28)	Moroccan-Spiced Fish Stew with Saffron (39), Mixed Greens with Golden Beets and Pomegranate Seeds (25)	Roasted Figs with Pomegranate Seeds and Mint (65)
25	Orange & Carrot Sunrise Smoothie with Turmeric (13)	Turkey & Sweet Potato Chili (45), Zucchini Noodles with Basil, Tomato & Garlic (33)	Miso-Marinated Sea Bass with Bok Choy (38), Romaine, Cucumber & Dill Salad with Olive Oil (25)	Cinnamon-Spiced Apple Bake with Walnuts (63)
26	Buckwheat & Berry Porridge with Coconut Milk (15)	Spiced Beef & Lentil Casserole (53), Lentil & Quinoa Salad with Roasted Red Peppers (27)	Broiled Tuna Steaks with Mango Salsa (39), Watercress & Pear Salad with Hazelnuts (26)	Anti-Inflammatory Lemon & Ginger Bars (67)
27	Avocado & Kiwi Anti-Inflammatory Smoothie (14)	Coconut-Curry Turkey Meatballs (46), Barley & Mushroom Risotto (30)	White Fish & Sweet Potato Coconut Stew (41), Endive & Walnut Salad with Pomegranate Dressing (26)	Matcha & Coconut Bliss Balls with Almonds (68)
28	Oatmeal with Turmeric, Cinnamon & Apples (17)	Roasted Venison with Garlic & Thyme (50), Turmeric-Spiced Bulgur with Mixed Herbs (32)	Anti-Inflammatory Steamed Mussels with Garlic (37), Romaine, Cucumber & Dill Salad with Olive Oil (25)	Golden Milk Popsicles with Coconut Cream (66)

Shopping List 22-28 Days

Fruits and Vegetables

◊ Green apples – 2

◊ Pears – 3

◊ Mango – 3

◊ Fresh pineapple – 1 medium

◊ Kiwi – 2

◊ Oranges – 2

◊ Fresh cherries – 1/2 cup

◊ Fresh figs – 4

◊ Lemons – 4

◊ Limes – 2

◊ Fresh pomegranate (or pomegranate seeds) – 1

◊ Fresh spinach – 2 cups

◊ Carrots – 6 medium

◊ Sweet potatoes – 4 medium

◊ Zucchini – 3 medium

◊ Fresh brussels sprouts – 1 lb

◊ Butternut squash – 1 small

◊ Romaine lettuce – 2 cups

◊ Cucumber – 2 medium

◊ Endive – 2 heads

◊ Mixed greens – 3 cups

◊ Golden beets – 2

◊ Fresh ginger – 3-inch piece

◊ Fresh parsley, thyme, basil, dill, cilantro, mint

Meat & Seafood

◊ Pork (for meatballs) – 1 lb

◊ Chicken thighs – 4 pieces (about 1 lb)

◊ Swordfish steaks – 2 pieces (about 1 lb)

◊ Cod fillets – 2 pieces (about 1 lb)

◊ Lamb chops – 2 pieces (about 1 lb)

◊ Halibut fillets – 2 pieces (about 1 lb)

◊ Sea bass fillets – 2 pieces (about 1 lb)

◊ Tuna steaks – 2 pieces (about 1 lb)

◊ Ground turkey – 1 lb

◊ Venison (or lean beef/pork) – 1 lb

◊ Mussels – 1 lb

General Shopping list for 28 Days

Grains, Pasta & Legumes

◊ Wild rice

◊ Quinoa

◊ Chickpea pasta

◊ Lentils

◊ Lentil pasta

◊ Quinoa pasta

◊ Farro

◊ Bulgur wheat

◊ Barley

◊ Millet

◊ Rolled oats

◊ Buckwheat

◊ Golden farro

Nuts & Seeds

◊ Pecans,Walnuts,Almonds,Hazelnuts ,Cashews

◊ Hemp seeds

◊ Chia seeds

◊ Shredded coconut

Canned & Packaged Goods

◊ Coconut cream

◊ Miso paste

◊ Maple syrup

◊ Olive oil

◊ Dijon mustard

◊ Honey

◊ Soy sauce

Baking & Miscellaneous

◊ Almond flour

◊ Coconut flour

◊ Rolled oats

◊ Pomegranate molasses

◊ Parchment paper

◊ Matcha powder

Dairy & Alternatives

◊ Almond milk (or preferred non-dairy milk)

◊ Coconut milk

◊ Eggs – 4

DON'T FORGET TO DRINK WATER

◊ The recommended daily water intake for the body is 1.5 to 2.5 liters.

◊ It is important to drink most of the water in the first half of the day and reduce the amount in the evening to avoid swelling.

◊ To help remind yourself to drink water, keep it always within sight, such as placing a cup of water on your work desk.

◊ When you go outside, always take a bottle of water with you.

◊ This way, you will gradually get used to drinking clean water, which is essential for the proper functioning of the entire body.

Ginger drink.

Water with ginger is part of the daily water intake. For 1.5 to 2 liters of water, add a few slices of ginger, half a lemon, and mint for aroma, if desired.

Ginger tea.

Brew green tea and grated ginger together. After the tea is brewed, add lemon. Find the perfect proportion of ingredients for yourself. The more ginger, the better, but remember, we shouldn't force ourselves to drink a bitter beverage. We are learning to eat healthily and with pleasure.

You should remember that the Ginger drink it's a water and the Ginger tea it's a tea.

For convenience, it's better to use water tracker apps on your phone or set reminders.

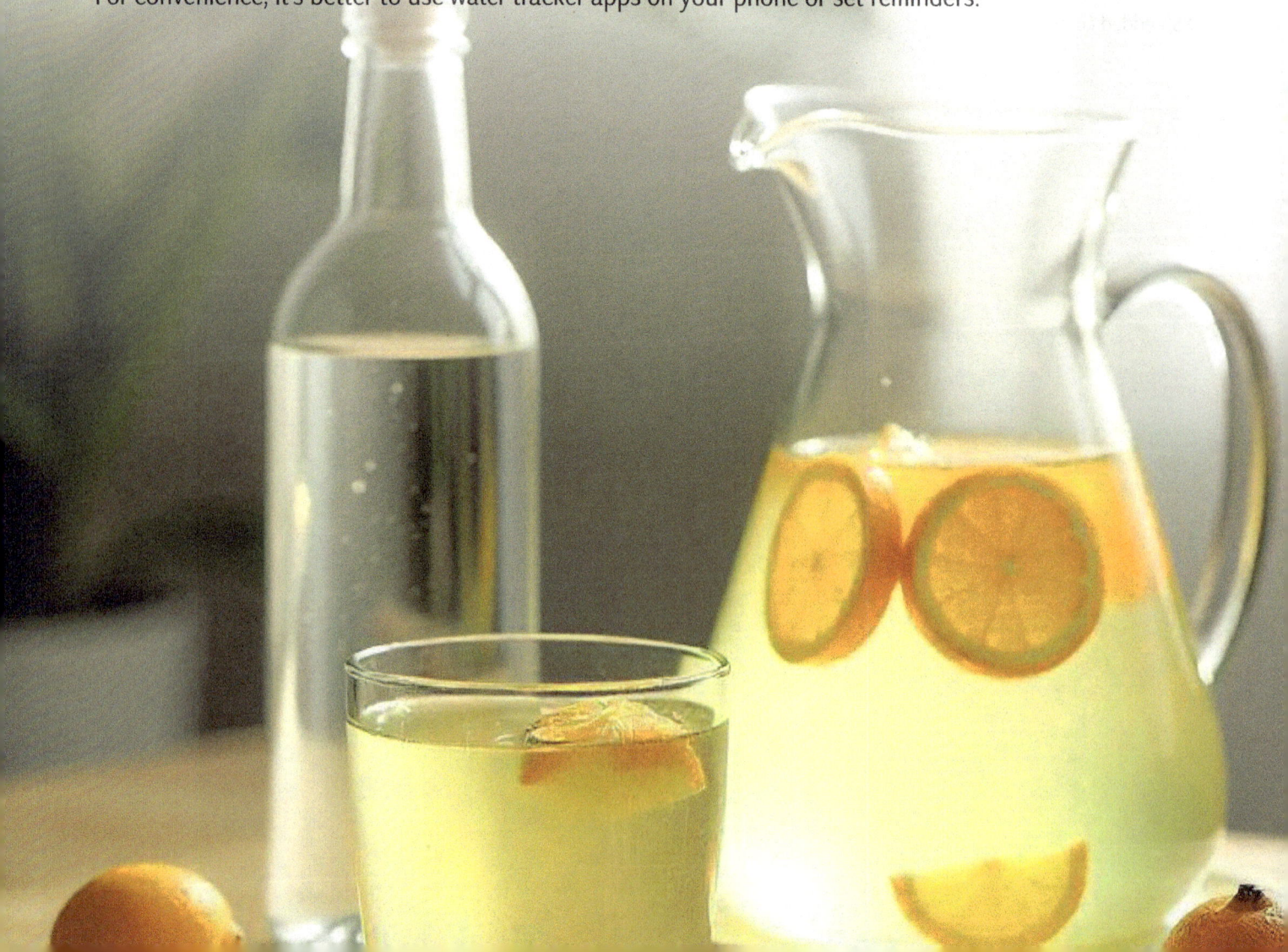

NATURE'S ANTI-INFLAMMATORY BENEFITS

A

- **Almonds:** Rich in vitamin E, healthy fats, and antioxidants, almonds support heart health, reduce inflammation, and protect against chronic diseases

- **Almond Butter:** A source of healthy fats, protein, and vitamin E, almond butter has anti-inflammatory properties and supports heart health

- **Almond Flour:** A gluten-free flour alternative that is high in healthy fats, fiber, and vitamin E, which is known for its antioxidant properties

- **Almond Milk:** A dairy-free alternative that is lower in calories and may contain vitamin E, an antioxidant that helps combat inflammation.

- **Amaranth:** A gluten-free grain rich in protein, fiber, and antioxidants. It contains anti-inflammatory compounds and is high in magnesium, which can help reduce inflammation in the body.

- **Apples:** Rich in fiber and antioxidants, apples help reduce inflammation, support digestive health, and improve heart health

- **Apple Cider Vinegar:** Known for its anti-inflammatory properties, apple cider vinegar helps balance the body's pH and supports digestion

- **Artichokes:** High in antioxidants and fiber, supporting liver health and digestion, which may aid in reducing inflammation.

- **Avocado:** High in monounsaturated fats, fiber, and antioxidants, avocados help reduce inflammation and support heart health

B

- **Balsamic Vinegar:** Contains polyphenols, antioxidants that help fight inflammation, protect cells, and reduce oxidative stress.

- **Banana:** Provides potassium, which supports heart health and muscle function. Its natural sweetness balances the earthy flavor of matcha.

- **Barley:** High in beta-glucan, barley supports heart health, stabilizes blood sugar, and promotes gut health, all of which are key in reducing inflammation.

- **Basil:** Known for its anti-inflammatory and antioxidant properties, basil helps protect cells and boost immunity.

- **Beef:** Grass-fed beef is a good source of high-quality protein, omega-3 fatty acids, and iron, all of which are essential for overall health. It helps support muscle mass and provides B-vitamins that aid in energy production.

- **Berries:** Rich in antioxidants, particularly anthocyanins, berries help reduce oxidative stress and inflammation, contributing to overall health and protection against chronic diseases.

- **Black Beans:** Packed with protein, fiber, and antioxidants, black beans support heart health and stabilize blood sugar levels.

- **Black Pepper:** Black pepper contains piperine, which enhances the bioavailability of curcumin in turmeric, making this combination even more effective in reducing inflammation.

- **Blackberries:** These berries are rich in antioxidants, particularly anthocyanins, which have anti-inflammatory properties. They also contain fiber, vitamin C, and manganese, which support overall immune health and help combat oxidative stress.

- **Blueberries:** High in antioxidants, especially anthocyanins, which help reduce oxidative stress and inflammation. Blueberries support brain health and cardiovascular health.

- **Broccoli:** High in vitamins K and C, fiber, and sulforaphane, broccoli has anti-inflammatory and anti-cancer properties.

- **Brown Rice:** A fiber-rich whole grain that stabilizes blood sugar and provides antioxidants to help reduce inflammation.

- **Brussels Sprouts:** Brussels sprouts are cruciferous vegetables, high in fiber, vitamins C and K, and antioxidants. The fiber aids in digestion and helps regulate blood sugar levels, while the antioxidants protect against oxidative stress, reducing inflammation in the body.

- **Brussels Sprouts:** High in vitamins C and K, Brussels sprouts contain glucosinolates, which may help lower the risk of inflammation-related diseases.

- **Buckwheat:** A gluten-free whole grain rich in fiber and antioxidants, buckwheat helps regulate blood sugar levels and supports heart health, contributing to reduced inflammation.

- **Bulgur:** A whole grain rich in fiber, bulgur supports digestion and helps maintain stable blood sugar levels, reducing inflammation.

- **Butter Lettuce:** This leafy green is rich in vitamins A and K, providing antioxidants that can help lower inflammation and support immune function.

- **Butternut Squash:** Rich in beta-carotene and fiber, butternut squash helps fight oxidative stress, supports gut health, and boosts the immune system, all of which contribute to reducing inflammation.

C

- **Cabbage**: Packed with fiber and antioxidants, cabbage helps detoxify the body, supports digestion, and may reduce the risk of chronic diseases.

- **Cacao Nibs:** Cacao nibs are high in antioxidants, magnesium, and fiber. They offer a crunchy texture and are known to promote heart health, improve mood, and reduce inflammation.

- **Capers:** These small buds are rich in antioxidants and have anti-inflammatory effects. They also add a tangy flavor that enhances the overall taste of the dip.

- **Carrots:** Carrots are rich in beta-carotene, a powerful antioxidant that helps reduce inflammation, supports immune health, and promotes healthy vision.
- **Cashew Butter:** Adds a creamy texture and provides magnesium and healthy fats, which support brain and heart health.
- **Cashews:** A good source of healthy fats, protein, and minerals like magnesium, cashews are beneficial for heart health and have anti-inflammatory properties.
- **Cauliflower & Broccoli:** These cruciferous vegetables are rich in sulforaphane, which has been shown to reduce inflammation and support liver detoxification.
- **Cauliflower:** A cruciferous vegetable, cauliflower contains antioxidants and fiber which help combat inflammation and support digestion.
- **Cayenne Pepper:** Contains capsaicin, which not only adds heat but also has anti-inflammatory effects by reducing pain and inflammation.
- **Celery:** Contains antioxidants and anti-inflammatory compounds, and its high water content helps detoxify and hydrate the body.
- **Cherry Tomatoes:** High in lycopene, cherry tomatoes help combat inflammation and are an excellent source of vitamins C and K. Rich in lycopene, an antioxidant linked to reduced inflammation and chronic disease prevention.
- **Chia Seeds:** Rich in omega-3 fatty acids, which have anti-inflammatory benefits, and high in fiber to support digestive health.
- **Chicken:** A lean source of protein, chicken is low in saturated fat and a great option for supporting muscle health. The high-quality protein helps repair and build tissues, reducing inflammation and promoting overall wellness.
- **Cilantro:** Contains antioxidants and phytonutrients that help reduce inflammation, promote detoxification, and improve digestion.
- **Cinnamon:** Contains compounds like cinnamaldehyde, which have potent anti-inflammatory effects, helping to reduce the risk of chronic diseases and inflammation.
- **Citrus Fruits:** High in vitamin C and flavonoids, citrus fruits can help reduce oxidative stress and inflammation in the body.
- **Cocoa:** Rich in flavonoids, which may help reduce inflammation and improve cardiovascular health.
- **Coconut Cream:** High in healthy fats, especially medium-chain triglycerides (MCTs), coconut cream helps reduce inflammation and supports gut and heart health.
- **Coconut Milk:** Contains healthy fats, particularly medium-chain triglycerides (MCTs), which can help reduce inflammation and improve metabolism.
- **Coconut Oil:** Contains medium-chain triglycerides (MCTs) that have anti-inflammatory and antioxidant effects.
- **Coconut:** The healthy fats in coconut provide anti-inflammatory benefits, as well as support for heart health and brain function.

- **Cod:** A lean source of protein and rich in vitamins and minerals like vitamin B12 and selenium, cod supports heart health, brain function, and immune system performance.
- **Cranberries:** Rich in antioxidants and anti-inflammatory compounds, cranberries support heart health and may help lower blood pressure.
- **Cumin and Coriander:** Both cumin and coriander have anti-inflammatory properties and aid digestion. They also help to detoxify the body and support the immune system.
- **Curry Powder:** Typically includes spices like cumin, coriander, and turmeric, which have anti-inflammatory properties and can enhance metabolism.

D

- **Dark Chocolate (70% or higher):** Packed with antioxidants, dark chocolate is known for its anti-inflammatory properties. The flavonoids in dark chocolate help improve blood circulation, protect heart health, and reduce oxidative stress.
- **Dijon Mustard:** Adds flavor while contributing a small amount of antioxidants and compounds that support digestion.
- **Dill:** Contains antioxidants and has been shown to have mild anti-inflammatory effects, in addition to providing vitamins A and C.
- **Duck Breast:** A rich source of protein, B-vitamins, and healthy fats. Duck meat is also high in iron, which supports the body's energy levels and immune system.

E

- **Edamame:** High in plant-based protein and fiber, edamame contains isoflavones that have anti-inflammatory properties.
- **Eggplant:** Rich in antioxidants like nasunin, which protects cells from oxidative stress and inflammation. It's also a good source of fiber, supporting gut health and reducing inflammation.
- **Eggs:** A great source of high-quality protein and healthy fats, providing essential nutrients without added sugars or unhealthy additives.
- **Endive:** Low in calories and high in fiber, endive is a great source of antioxidants that can help reduce inflammation and support digestive health.

F

- **Farro:** This ancient grain is high in fiber, protein, and essential nutrients like magnesium and B vitamins. Its complex carbohydrates help maintain steady blood sugar levels and reduce inflammation.
- **Fennel:** Contains fiber, vitamin C, and potassium, which aid in digestion, immune function, and inflammation reduction.
- **Feta Cheese:** Optional, but if used, provides a source of calcium and protein. Choose a lower-fat version to keep the dish lighter.

> **Figs**: High in fiber, vitamins, and antioxidants, figs support digestive health and have been linked to reduced inflammation. They are also a natural source of sweetness.

> **Flaxseed**: A source of omega-3 fatty acids and fiber, flaxseed can help reduce inflammation and support heart health.

G

> **Garlic**: Allicin, a compound in garlic, has been shown to reduce inflammation and support the immune system.

> **Ginger:** Contains gingerol, a compound that has strong anti-inflammatory properties and helps reduce muscle pain, joint pain, and general inflammation.

> **Golden Beets**: Rich in betalains, golden beets possess antioxidant and anti-inflammatory properties that can help combat oxidative stress and inflammation in the body.

> **Grapefruit**: A great source of vitamin C and flavonoids, grapefruit is known to support immune function and combat oxidative stress.

> **Grass-Fed Beef**: A lean protein source, grass-fed beef is high in omega-3 fatty acids, which help reduce inflammation. It also provides essential nutrients like iron and B vitamins.

> **Greek Yogurt:** Rich in probiotics and protein, yogurt supports gut health and contributes to reducing inflammation by fostering a healthy microbiome.

> **Green Olives**: Rich in monounsaturated fats and antioxidants, olives have anti-inflammatory properties and promote heart health. They also contain vitamin E, which helps protect cells from oxidative damage.

> **Ground Turkey:** A lean source of protein, turkey is low in fat and packed with amino acids that support muscle health, tissue repair, and immune function. It's a great option for an anti-inflammatory diet because it's easy on digestion and doesn't contain the saturated fats found in red meats.

H

> **Halibut:** A lean fish high in protein and low in fat, halibut is rich in B vitamins, including vitamin B12, which support brain health and energy production. Halibut also provides a good amount of selenium, a powerful antioxidant that helps fight inflammation.

> **Hazelnuts**: Packed with healthy fats, fiber, and vitamin E, hazelnuts are known for their anti-inflammatory properties and can help improve heart health.

> **Hemp Seeds:** Rich in omega-3 and omega-6 fatty acids, hemp seeds provide essential fatty acids to further support heart and brain health.

> **Honey:** A natural sweetener with anti-inflammatory effects, honey can help soothe the digestive system and promote healing.

> **Hummus**: Made primarily from chickpeas, hummus is high in protein and fiber, which can help reduce inflammation. Chickpeas contain anti-inflammatory compounds and are rich in vitamins and minerals.

K

> **Kale**: High in vitamins A, C, and K, kale is an excellent anti-inflammatory food. It also has calcium and fiber that support bone health and digestion.

> **Kidney Beans**: High in fiber, which supports gut health, and rich in antioxidants that combat inflammation.

L

> **Lamb**: High in protein, iron, and B vitamins, which support immune health and muscle function. Choosing lean cuts of lamb helps reduce saturated fat intake, aligning with anti-inflammatory principles.

> **Lean Beef**: A great source of high-quality protein and iron. Reducing fat intake helps avoid inflammation that can be caused by saturated fats.

> **Lean Beef:** A great source of high-quality protein, lean beef is also rich in iron, zinc, and B vitamins, which are essential for maintaining a healthy immune system and reducing inflammation. Opting for lean cuts helps minimize the intake of unhealthy fats.

> **Lemon**: High in vitamin C, lemons are potent antioxidants that help support the immune system, fight free radicals, and reduce inflammation.

> **Lentils**: High in fiber and protein, lentils help to reduce blood sugar levels and contain polyphenols, which have anti-inflammatory properties.

M

> **Mackerel:** Mackerel is rich in omega-3 fatty acids, especially EPA and DHA, which are known for their anti-inflammatory properties. These fats support heart, brain, and joint health, while reducing inflammation throughout the body.

> **Mango**: High in vitamins A and C, mangoes are loaded with antioxidants, which help fight free radicals and reduce inflammation. They also promote skin and digestive health.

> **Mango**: Packed with vitamins A and C, mangoes are rich in antioxidants and have anti-inflammatory properties that can support immune function and skin health.

> **Matcha**: A powdered green tea rich in catechins, which are potent antioxidants that help reduce inflammation and protect cells from damage.

> **Microgreens**: These tiny greens are packed with vitamins C, E, and K, and are rich in antioxidants, which can help lower inflammation and improve immune function.

> **Millet**: A gluten-free grain that is high in fiber, protein, and magnesium. Its low glycemic index helps regulate blood sugar levels, reducing inflammation.

> **Miso:** A fermented soybean paste rich in probiotics that support gut health, immune function, and overall digestive wellness. Miso also contains antioxidants that combat oxidative stress.

- **Mixed Greens**: High in vitamins A, C, and K, mixed greens provide antioxidants that can help reduce inflammation and boost overall health.
- **Mushrooms**: Known for their immune-boosting properties, mushrooms contain polysaccharides and antioxidants that reduce inflammation.

N

- **Nutritional Yeast**: A source of B vitamins and protein, nutritional yeast adds a cheesy flavor while contributing to overall nutrient density.
- **Nuts**: Rich in healthy fats, fiber, and protein, walnuts and pecans contain antioxidants that combat inflammation.

O

- **Oats:** Provide fiber that helps regulate blood sugar and supports gut health, both crucial for reducing inflammation.
- **Olive Oil**: Extra virgin olive oil is a key component of the Mediterranean diet and contains healthy fats and antioxidants that can reduce inflammation.
- **Oregano:** This herb has **antioxidant** and **anti-inflammatory** properties, thanks to compounds like rosmarinic acid. It supports immune function and helps reduce inflammation in the body.

P

- **Paprika**: Rich in antioxidants, particularly carotenoids, paprika can help reduce oxidative stress and inflammation in the body.
- **Parsley:** Contains vitamins A, C, and K and has natural anti-inflammatory properties.
- **Pears**: High in dietary fiber, particularly pectin, which helps to promote gut health. Pears also contain antioxidants that combat oxidative stress.
- **Pecans**: Packed with healthy fats, protein, and antioxidants, pecans can help reduce oxidative stress and inflammation in the body.
- **Peppers:** High in vitamin C and antioxidants, which help protect cells from damage and inflammation
- **Pineapple:** Contains bromelain, an enzyme that reduces inflammation and supports digestion. It's also packed with vitamin C, which helps strengthen the immune system.
- **Pomegranate Seeds**: These seeds are packed with antioxidants, particularly punicalagins, which have been shown to reduce inflammation and improve heart health.
- **Pork**: A good source of lean protein, iron, and zinc, supporting muscle function and immune health. Choosing a lean cut helps reduce saturated fats.
- **Pumpkin Seeds**: Loaded with magnesium, zinc, and antioxidants, pumpkin seeds are known for their anti-inflammatory properties and heart health benefits.

- **Pumpkin**: Rich in vitamins A and C, antioxidants, and fiber, pumpkin helps lower inflammation and supports immune function.
- **Purple Cabbage:** Contains anthocyanins and vitamins C and K, which help reduce inflammation and oxidative stress.

Q

- **Quinoa Pasta**: A gluten-free option rich in plant-based protein, fiber, and essential amino acids, which help reduce inflammation and maintain blood sugar stability.
- **Quinoa**: A complete protein containing all essential amino acids, quinoa is also rich in magnesium, which helps reduce inflammation.

R

- **Radishes**: Known for their high fiber content and antioxidants, radishes can support digestive health and may help to reduce inflammation in the body.
- **Raspberries**: Packed with antioxidants, vitamins C and E, which combat inflammation.
- **Red cabbage**: High in antioxidants like vitamin C, which helps reduce oxidative stress and inflammation in the body.
- **Red Onion**: Contains quercetin, an antioxidant that may help to reduce inflammation and lower the risk of chronic diseases.
- **Romaine Lettuce**: Low in calories and high in vitamins A and K, Romaine lettuce is hydrating and provides antioxidants that may help reduce inflammation.
- **Rosemary**: Contains compounds that may help reduce inflammation and has antioxidant properties

S

- **Saffron**: Known for its anti-inflammatory properties, saffron also acts as a mood booster and has antioxidant effects.
- **Sage**: Contains powerful antioxidants like rosmarinic acid, which has anti-inflammatory effects. Sage also aids digestion.
- **Salmon:** A rich source of omega-3 fatty acids, which help reduce inflammation and support heart and brain health. Omega-3s also contribute to healthier skin and improved mood.
- **Scallops:** These are a rich source of lean protein and omega-3 fatty acids, which are beneficial for heart health and help to reduce inflammation. Scallops also provide essential minerals like selenium and magnesium, which support immune function and muscle health.
- **Sea Bass:** A high-quality source of lean protein and omega-3 fatty acids, which are crucial for reducing inflammation, supporting brain health, and maintaining heart health.
- **Sesame Oil**: Contains sesamol, an antioxidant that combats oxidative stress and inflammation in the body.
- **Shredded Coconut**: Provides healthy fats and fiber, which help reduce inflammation and support heart health.

> **Shrimp**: A lean source of protein and omega-3 fatty acids, shrimp is excellent for reducing inflammation and supporting heart health.

> **Smoked Paprika**: Adds a smoky flavor along with antioxidant compounds like capsaicin, which may help reduce inflammation.

> **Spinach:** High in antioxidants, particularly vitamins A and C, spinach helps reduce oxidative stress and inflammation. It's also rich in fiber, which supports digestive health.

> **Steel-Cut Oats**: High in soluble fiber, which can help reduce cholesterol and inflammation. They are also rich in antioxidants and beneficial for heart health.

> **Strawberries**: Packed with antioxidants and vitamin C, strawberries help combat inflammation and support immune health.

> **Sun-Dried Tomatoes**: High in lycopene, an antioxidant that supports heart health and may lower inflammation levels.

> **Sweet Potato:** High in beta-carotene and antioxidants, sweet potatoes help reduce inflammation, support immune function, and promote gut health due to their fiber content.

> **Swordfish:** A lean protein source rich in selenium, omega-3 fatty acids, and vitamin D, which support anti-inflammatory processes and heart health.

T

> **Tahini**: Made from sesame seeds, tahini contains healthy fats and polyphenols that combat inflammation.

> **Tart Cherries**: Rich in anthocyanins, tart cherries have strong anti-inflammatory properties. They are known to reduce muscle soreness and improve recovery after exercise. Tart cherry juice has also been shown to lower markers of inflammation in the body.

> **Thyme**: Contains thymol, an essential oil with antioxidant and antimicrobial properties.

> **Tomatoes**: High in lycopene, which has been shown to reduce inflammation and promote heart health.

> **Trout:** A great source of omega-3 fatty acids and protein, trout supports heart health and reduces inflammation, benefiting brain and joint function.

> **Turkey:** A lean source of high-quality protein, turkey is rich in B-vitamins, particularly niacin and vitamin B6, which support metabolic and cardiovascular health.

> **Turmeric**: A potent anti-inflammatory spice, curcumin in turmeric helps reduce inflammation and support joint health.

W

> **Walnuts:** A great source of omega-3 fatty acids, walnuts help fight inflammation and support brain health.

> **Watercress:** This leafy green is rich in vitamins A, C, and K, along with antioxidants that help combat inflammation and promote heart health.

> **White Beans**: Rich in fiber and plant-based protein, white beans help reduce inflammation and support digestive health.

> **White Fish:** Provides high-quality protein and is low in saturated fat. It's a good source of omega-3 fatty acids, which help reduce inflammation and support heart health.

> **Whole Wheat Couscous**: A good source of fiber and protein, whole wheat couscous helps regulate blood sugar levels and supports digestive health.

> **Wild Rice**: A whole grain that is high in fiber and antioxidants, wild rice helps to reduce inflammation and improve digestion.

Z

> **Zucchini:** Rich in antioxidants like vitamin C and beta-carotene, zucchini adds anti-inflammatory nutrients to the dish and increases its fiber content.

Dear Readers,

I want to take a moment to express my deepest gratitude to each of you for picking up this book and making it a part of your journey toward better health and well-being. Writing The Ultimate Anti-Inflammatory Diet Cookbook for Beginners has been a labor of love, and knowing that it might help you in even the smallest way truly fills my heart with joy.

Every recipe, tip, and piece of advice in these pages comes from a place of genuine care and a desire to make a positive impact in your life. I poured my soul into this book, hoping it would inspire you, nourish your body, and bring more balance to your daily life.

As a token of my appreciation, I've included a special bonus for you—your very own Anti-Inflammatory Diet Tracker. This tracker is not just a tool; it's your companion on this journey to better health. You can print it out and use it daily to monitor your meals, energy levels, physical activity, and how your body responds to the foods you eat.

Tracking your progress helps you stay focused and motivated. It allows you to see the changes, celebrate the victories, and make adjustments when needed. Remember, this journey isn't about perfection—it's about progress and consistency. You deserve to feel your best every day, and I'm so excited for you to see the positive impact that making small, mindful choices can have on your life.

From the bottom of my heart, thank you for allowing me to be a part of your story. Here's to health, happiness, and the delicious moments we create along the way.

PLEASE LET ME KNOW HOW YOU LIKE IT!

Positive ratings, reviews and constructive suggestions from awesome people like you help others to feel confident about choosing this book and help us to continue providing great books.

Share your happy experience online in Amazon with the following three steps:

- Go to the product detail page of this book on Amazon
- Stroll down to Review this product section
- Click Write a customer review in the Customer Reviews section
- Select a Star Rating
- Scribble your happy thoughts, add photos and videos. Submit

Thank you in advance for your review ❤️

With gratitude,

Helga Grinley

Made in the USA
Monee, IL
14 July 2025